ALAN HUNTER D.Dt.

Allergies Make You Fat

ASHGROVE PRESS, BATH

First published in Great Britain by
AHGROVE PRESS LIMITED
7 Locksbrook Road Estate
Bath, Avon BA1 3DZ

ISBN 1 85398 077 3

Dedicated to my son and daughter
Alan and Nicola

Typeset in 11/12½ Compugraphic Palatino by
Action Typsetting Limited, Gloucester
Printed and bound in Great Britain by
Redwood Books Ltd., Trowbridge,
Wiltshire

CONTENTS

PART ONE
HOW TO DISCOVER YOUR FOOD ALLERGIES

PART TWO
WHAT TO DO ABOUT YOUR FOOD ALLERGIES

Acknowledgements

I wish to thank the following, either for their direct or indirect contribution to this book, or for their works which I have drawn upon in the preparation of the manuscript:

Charlotte Gerson, of the Gerson Institute in California, whose personal communications I have been delighted to receive.

Charlotte's father, Max Gerson M.D. whose dietary therapy has saved the lives of thousands. His work reaffirms my unshakeable belief in correct diet as a means of restoring health.

Sir Robert McCarrison whose fascinating work with the Hunzakuts still serves as the quintessential study of the link between diet and health.

Francis M. Pottenger Jr., M.D., who, along with McCarrison and Gerson, ranks as one of the giants in nutritional science.

Professor Arnold Ehret for his lucid and logical conclusions on fasting, diet and physiology.

Henry Lindlahr M.D., whose writings on natural therapeutics were ahead of his time.

Dr. Norman Walker, advocate of raw vegetable juices, who died recently, aged 110.

Dr. George Watson of California whose food allergy experiments in the late 1960's first led me to understand the critical relationship between everyday eating habits and ill health.

I wish also to thank the following for permission to quote: Gordon Allen of Carol Publishing Group, New York, for information from *The Pulse Test*; Beth Croteau of Avery Publishing, Wayne, New Jersey, for material from *Enzyme Nutrition*; Irene Harper of Churchill Livingstone, for deficiency tables from *Nutrition and its Disorders*; Howard Watson of

Random House, for *Goodbye to Arthritis;* Routledge (Unwin Hyman) London, for an excerpt from *Let's Get Well;* by Adelle Davis, Routledge for material from *Food Allergy* by Robert Woodward and Rita Green; and Dr J.L. Grant for assisting in a glossary.

Thanks also to Robin Campbell, my publisher, for his understanding and appreciation of the subject.

My son and daughter, Alan and Nicola, have played their part in encouraging me to the finishing line, so they too, have to be thanked.

PART I

How to Discover your Food Allergies

ONE

You're Not Fat, You're Allergic

I hope to explain to you that, contrary to everything you've ever been told about any weight problem you may have, it is not the calorie, or even the carbohydrate content of your diet that counts, but whether or not you are allergic to the foods that you are eating.

I would go as far as to say this small book contains the Dieter's Holy Grail – the true reason behind the widespread obesity and weight problems that beset our modern society.

The phenomenon of food allergies has exploded in the past 20 or so years, and they have been rightly linked to a vast variety of common health disorders such as arthritis and depression whose causes have hitherto baffled our doctors. This book goes further and points to food allergies as being responsible for your being overweight. It shows you how to test your own diet at home and pinpoint the culprit foods. By removing the foods to which you are allergic from your diet (the 'allergens') your body's metabolism will be corrected and your weight, whether it is presently over or under, will normalise.

You may well insist that you have no allergies; but believe me, if you are overweight, you will almost certainly be allergic to something in your diet.

As one of the first people in Britain to be tested for food allergies (albeit in Rome in 1972 by the old-fashioned 'sniff' tests) I certainly found out I was allergic to foods, whilst previously I would have said I had no allergies whatsoever. I had no runny nose, no sneezing or itching;

nothing that would be recognised as 'allergies'. But with food it can be a cunning and detective-like search that unravels the unsuspecting allergens that almost all of us have – whether we know it or not.

I work in Clinical Ecology, which, like osteopathy, herbalism, acupuncture and other 'alternative' disciplines is outside orthodox medical school training but which, because of its tremendous success in correcting chronic health problems, is attracting more and more medical doctors into its ranks.

Clinical Ecology is the relatively new discipline which looks for a link between health disorders and the patient's diet, or environment. It has had tremendous success in showing patients the true cause of disorders which their G.P.s have found particularly difficult to treat. Common complaints such as arthritis or disabling fatigue, for which doctors can offer no 'cure' other than prescribing palliative drugs, have often disappeared once problem foods were identified and removed from the patients' diets.

Symptoms of food/chemical allergies

Besides overweight – and underweight – an enormous diversity of symptoms can be produced by foods and/or chemicals. Although many doctors may show some surprise at the range of disorders which can be induced by so-called ordinary foods, the fact remains that these conditions can indeed be the result of ingesting common foodstuffs.

It is important to impress upon the reader that although the symptoms listed below can certainly be caused by food/chemical allergies, it is essential that your doctor examines you thoroughly so as to eliminate any other – and possibly more serious – causes:

Aggressiveness	Obesity	Poor Memory
Behaviour problems	Migraine	Diarrhoea
Irritability	Hyperactivity	Skin Disorders
Lack of Concentration	Phobias	Obsessions
Frequent Urination	Stammering	Broken Nails

Personality Changes	Receding gums	Blindness
Social Withdrawal	Flatulence	Bruising
Addictive behaviour	Palpitations	Mouth cracks
Argumentativeness	Nervousness	Constipation
'Bloodshot' cheeks	Asthma	Haemorrhoids
Schizophrenia	Infertility	Impotence
High Blood Pressure	Colitis	Swellings
Tinnitus	Bad Breath	Insomnia
Mouth Ulcers	Loss of Hair	Cramps
Loss of Humour	Poor Eyesight	Epilepsy
Menstrual Difficulties	Depression	Fatigue
Handwriting Variations	Itching	Alcoholism
Respiratory Trouble	Arthritis	Fibrositis

If you have never been tested for food allergies and you suffer from any of the above conditions, do not for a moment dismiss the probability of your diet being the cause; you will almost certainly never know if food is implicated until you have been tested.

From my own practice I can tell you that nearly *everyone* who has consulted me (very few knowing beforehand that they had food allergies) has shown some adverse activity in their pulse when challenged with food tests. You may have suffered for many years with one of the above symptoms yet never at any time considered a link with food. Prepare yourself for a surprise!

Our weight-controlling glands are affected by food allergies

The bodily imbalance which creates the overweight individual is a disturbed thyroid gland. Unwittingly, the fatty eats foods which are adversely affecting the thyroid – foods to which he or she is 'allergic'.

The hugely important thyroid gland is situated at the lower front of the neck, attached to the windpipe, and is the regulator of our metabolic rate – the speed at which our bodies 'burn up' food.

Needless to say, any malfunction in this gland's activities can have a disastrous effect on our weight.

A person with a slow metabolism will easily put on weight, will often feel sluggish and will have poor energy levels. And the simple, most often overlooked reason for this soul-destroying condition is that the thyroid can be dysfunctioning because the eater is unknowingly allergic to items in his diet.

If the gland malfunctions, it will produce less of the hormone thyroxine than is ideal for perfect metabolic activity. This results in overweight, with the sufferer feeling lethargic. Poor circulation and elimination are other consequences of a disturbed thyroid gland.

As with many imbalances and disorders within the body, there are degrees of malfunction. Symptoms such as respiratory symptoms, urinary system disorders and skin diseases will likely be present, with greater incidence or severity than among those people with satisfactory thyroid activity. Often anaemia is present and that is blamed for the low energy levels.

Disturbed thyroid functioning is much more common than many physicians realise, as most doctors are looking for full-blown symptoms. The fact is, many sufferers can have 'sub-clinical' symptoms which are not easily detectable, yet will indeed have poorly functioning thyroid glands, with the resultant fatigue and overweight.

Dr. Broda Barnes stated that no less than 40 percent of the adult population of the United States suffers from hypothyroidism – a probable underestimate according to Stephen Langer M.D., author of *Solved: The Riddle of Illness*, a book highlighting the condition and showing it to be far more common than hitherto considered. It is almost certain that a similar percentage of sufferers will exist in Great Britain, a country with a similarly appalling health record – and diet – to the U.S.

As well as hypothyroidism, the opposite side of the coin – hyperthyroidism – is probably more common than previously considered. It is simply another version of a disturbed thyroid gland. But this time the person may constantly rush around, hardly sitting still, apparently full of energy, but all the time getting thinner and more and more highly-strung. Again this condition can often be overlooked by the G.P.

This thin-as-a-rake person, who can eat anything and not put on weight, will be eating foods to which his thyroid gland is reacting – but in the opposite way to that in which the fatty reacts.

The thin person will have a fast metabolism because of the extra thyroxine pouring from his malfunctioning thyroid gland. If he tests himself for food allergens and removes the culprit foods, his metabolism will normalise and his struggle to *gain* weight will be over, as his weight corrects itself.

Whether the allergenic foods responsible for disturbing the thyroid are influencing its function directly, or indirectly via the brain, we are not quite sure.

That the brain is influenced in food allergic reactions is beyond question; migraine and depression, both typical food allergy symptoms, are good examples. As impulses from the brain are responsible for the releasing of hormones from our glands into the bloodstream,[1] it is quite possible that these very impulses are interfered with by these allergenic foods, so influencing adversely the hormone release from the thyroid.

When your thyroid gland malfunctions, it can have an adversely-influencing effect on the other endocrine glands, such as the pituitary, so by normalising the thyroid function, this will have a knock-on, stabilising effect throughout your system.

By testing for food allergens, and removing them from your diet, the normalising of your entire system will take place, and amongst the health benefits that will come your way, besides the delightful, confidence-boosting element of weight loss and all the joys that automatically follow, will be better health and hopefully the removal of any other annoying little symptoms.

How I made the Allergy/Thyroid Discovery

About eighteen months ago I decided to test myself for low thyroid activity – hypothyroidism – merely out of curiosity. It has been shown that the most accurate method of diagnosing an under-active thyroid is by means of the Barnes Basal Temperature Test,[2] named after Dr. Broda Barnes, a clinical researcher in hypothyroidism for over half a century. The simple under-arm test has been shown to be far superior to hospital tests for assessing thyroid function. It consists of taking your under-arm temperature for two consecutive mornings. Women can obtain the most accurate reading when menstruating, on the second or third day after your period starts.

If your average reading is below 97.8 deg F. then low thyroid activity is indicated.[3]

The normal (basal) temperature range is 97.8 deg. F to 98.2 deg. F. When the thyroid output is low, the temperature tends to fluctuate, whilst generally remaining below 97.8 deg. F. The metabolic rate changes about ten percent for each degree of temperature. A low basal temperature indicates a slow metabolic rate whilst a high temperature implies a fast rate.

One morning, following a day of eating foods to which I knew I was allergic, my morning reading was 97.2 deg. That day and the following three days I behaved myself and stuck to an allergen-free diet. On the second morning my temperature showed 97.4 deg.: creeping up, I thought. On the third morning it increased again – it was 97.5 deg. F. And on the fourth morning it had gone up once more – to 97.55. It was showing daily improvement. Then, on the fourth day, at night, I stupidly broke the diet when I was invited out to a social gathering.

The following morning, I took the temperature as usual, not expecting for a moment that anything special would show. But it most certainly did. It had dropped dramatically down to the figure it had been on day 1 – 97.2 deg! I was baffled. I couldn't work it out for a while, until it finally dawned on me. I was witnessing the very explanation of a particular phenomenon that Clinical Ecologists recognised happened, but could not explain.

Patients who consulted Clinical Ecologists for their health problems found that, when the problem foods were identified and removed from their diets, as well as often losing their distressing symptoms, if they were overweight, their weight would also normalise.

It was not known what physiological process was involved in this wonderful bonus. Some practitioners considered that, as these ill patients were recommended to go onto a healthy diet anyway, it was this mere improvement in their eating habits which achieved the weight loss. Others acknowledged that the removal of food allergens resulted in weight loss, but none was able to explain the mechanism behind it.

My temperature-taking had however supplied me with just that explanation. My thyroid function was being adversely affected by allergenic foods, creating a slow metabolism with, amongst other symptoms, its resultant overweight.

I kept eating allergenic foods for that day, just to see what would happen the following morning. Amazingly, it dropped even further – to 97.00 deg. I was delighted, because it was further confirmation of my original thinking.

After a few days, during which the findings preyed constantly on my mind, I decided on another experiment. I had reached the results above by first eating 'safe' foods, then consuming allergenic substances. What would happen if I fasted for five days, eating absolutely nothing, making me super-sensitive to all foods when eating recommenced? It would be a better, more valid test, I thought, than the first.

For five days I ate nothing whatsoever, but drank bottled water (it is not as heroic as you may think; you lose all sense of hunger after 48 hours on a fast!).

During these five days, and as expected, each morning's temperature showed a slight increase. On the fifth evening I ate potatoes – to which I knew I was allergic. The following morning's temperature should dramatically drop if my theory was correct. It did. It dropped to the reading prior to the fast. Proof again, if need be, I thought.

But just in case it could be said that it had been the mere consumption of food – any food, regardless of whether I was allergic to it or not – that had made the reading drop, I decided on one final test.

After a few days of 'bad' eating, to maintain a good run of low readings, I went on another five day fast. Each morning, again, my temperature slowly rose, and on the fifth evening I ate loads of grapes and apples – foods to which I knew I was NOT allergic. If again my theory was to stand up, the following morning's temperature reading should increase slightly. It did. I stayed on apples and grapes that day and added pears, another food to which I was not allergic. The following morning it had increased yet again!

That was the conclusive evidence I wanted and which was the inspiration for this book – something that would give people with life-long weight problems a real explanation as to why they can gain weight from seemingly modest amounts of food.

One may well ask, why hasn't such an important dietary tool as weight loss by food allergy detection been more widely used before? Simply because the allergy link to common disorders is relatively – in medical terms – new, and you have to consider that only a few years ago nutritional scientists had discovered only a hundred or so enzymes. Now, a mere few years later, they have discovered thousands more, and the list is still growing! Nutrition is a relatively new science; and food allergies (Clinical Ecology) even newer.

It is only in the last couple of decades that awareness of the food allergy concept has spread. People all over the world have been testing their diets and discovering they had food allergies of which they were totally unaware. And, more importantly, they have found that health disorders of many years' standing, and which had resisted orthodox medical treatment, were clearing up once the offending foodstuffs were removed from their diet.

This book is another step in the food allergy revolution: the discovery that we are fat because some of the items in our diet are directly influencing – adversely – the function of our weight-controlling thyroid gland and that, by avoiding these foods, our metabolism will be corrected and our weight will normalise.

The wonderful, unique bonus with the food allergy approach to weight management is that you may well be able to eat foods which you previously considered would be fattening – as long as you prove not to be allergic to them. Chips, and indeed even white sugar – although not recommended for obvious health reasons – have been eaten *without restriction* by overweight patients who would still lose weight beautifully, simply because they proved not to be allergic to these items!

This absolutely unique approach, which can allow the overweight individual to lose weight whilst eating without restriction such a 'fattening' food as white sugar, and the ever-thin individual to gain weight by the same method, marks a monumental step forward in weight management study. This twin-strike dietary approach demands to be treated with the highest respect.

The removal of the food allergens within your diet will not only return your weight to normal, probably for the first time in many years, but you may well notice any niggly little symptoms which you have learned to live with over the years, disappearing as a result of your dietary change.

Clinical Ecologists treat patients by uncovering environmental and dietary causes for their illnesses, so whenever I refer to diet in this book, I mean anything that goes into your mouth or body; food of any kind, water in any form, alcohol, tobacco smoke and other inhalants such as car exhaust fumes or chemical hair sprays; even the air that you breathe. So if I suggest that car exhaust fumes, or the gum on the back of postage stamps, are part of your diet, I hope you will understand my good intentions!

The vast majority of overweight people – if not every single one of them – can be made slim by this approach. It explains too, why your friend can eat high calorie meals without putting on an ounce, yet if you try the same, you balloon. The difference between you and her is that she is not allergic to the foods on the menu whilst you are.

Or it could be, that she *is* allergic to foods in her diet, but they are affecting her thyroid in the opposite manner to how your's reacts; her metabolic rate runs off at a gallop whilst your's slows down almost to a grinding halt!

This food allergy approach examines your body's reaction to each food substance and determines whether that food is responsible for your weight problem.

Weight loss link to food allergies

Clinical Ecologists, many of them medical doctors, have noticed some connection between food allergies and weight correction, but until now no-one has identified the exact process.

In *The Pulse Test*,[4] Arthur F. Coca M.D. states 'There is now convincing evidence that many cases of overweight are due to food allergy, and that when the food allergens are withdrawn from the diet the weight falls to the normal level for the individual, and remains there *without any restriction of the safe foods, including starches, sugars and fats.*

He cites one lady, a Miss M., who, as well as suffering from migraine, was plagued by overweight. After removing the foods to which she was allergic, not only did her migraine disappear but her weight reduced to normal and all the while she was able to eat to her appetite's content of potatoes and sugar, amongst other non-allergenic foods.

Another patient, a Mrs P. who was over 70, was also overweight. She lost 15lbs in weight by avoiding her allergic foods. Although she was allergic to corn, she could eat other cereals without restriction. And amongst the other foods that she could indulge in to her heart's content were potatoes and again, sugar! Remember too, that every reducing diet in existence warns you strictly to avoid such food as sugar.

Another of Coca's patients, a Mrs B., proved allergic to cow's milk, citrus fruit, carrot, beet-spinach, asparagus, onion and nuts. She lost two and a half stone, with again, no ban whatsoever against the 'fattening' starches and sweets. Not only did she lose all that weight, but she totally recovered from her depression as well as all her other symptoms.

Dr. John Mansfield[5] found that treating patients for food allergy also produced some magnificent weight losses. One woman lost 7lbs in 6 days, another 8½lbs in 5½ days, and a man 1 stone in 6 days!

In *'Minerals: Kill or Cure?'*, the authors[6] report on a man who weighed 300lbs. but who, when salt was omitted from his diet, lost 10lbs. in weight in one day! A case of salt allergy I ask?

One of Coca's patients was a chap who was 25lbs UNDERweight, with a disturbingly high blood pressure of 180/108. In six weeks, after eliminating the allergenic foods from his diet, the patient's blood pressure was down to 128/78 and he had GAINED almost a stone!

Rita Greer and Robert Woodward, in their book *Food Allergy,*[7] have this to say about the connection between obesity and food allergies: 'People have been puzzled by either not losing weight when going on a low calorie diet and then being successful when adopting a diet of normal calorific content but which merely excludes particular foods – their obesity being caused by food allergy, not by excess of calories! All slimmers' diets are to some extent elimination diets but do not give lasting results because as soon as you return to your previous diet you can start ingesting the allergens responsible for your obesity once more!'

Patricia Byrivers, in *Goodbye to Arthritis*, with a foreword by Dr. Patrick Kingsley of the British Society for Nutritional Medicine,[8] talking of people who have food allergies, says: 'The first bonus which usually arises after allergic people eliminate their allergies ... is that they start to lose weight. It does not seem to make any difference if chips and sweets are eaten, as long as you are not allergic to them.'

Further evidence that obesity is a food allergy factor comes from a study in which digestive enzymes were employed to help allergic individuals.

Treating allergy-based conditions with large doses of digestive enzymes in this study showed superb clinical improvements. The details of the study[9] are shown below

Table 2

Number of cases	% Improved
34 Bronchial Asthma	88
12 Food Asthma	92
42 Food Eczema	83
19 Hay Fever	80
11 Loose Bowels	100
54 Normal Weight	Remained Constant
29 Overweight	93
197 Underweight	91
29 Urticaria or Hives	86

in Table 2. And as you will see, when overweight people were given digestive enzymes in order to clear up their allergic symptoms, 93 percent of them reduced weight. And, not only that, but those people who were underweight showed a 91 percent normalisation of their weight, whilst the normal-weight patient stayed at his normal weight! This is further evidence that obesity is inextricably linked to food allergies.[10]

The above study was carried out by a Dr. Sansum who suggested that food allergy appeared to be due, in part, to absorption of incompletely digested protein molecules. Remember, that was back in 1932!

TWO

Food and Chemical Allergies As A Widespread Phenomenon

Allergy means 'Altered reaction'.

The majority of food allergic persons will never know that they have food allergies, for a number of reasons. Firstly, as they often consume the culprit foods extremely regularly, no clear link will emerge between any symptoms and a particular food; secondly, the foods can cause reactions within the body (such as adverse thyroid activity) which are unlikely to be evident to the eater.

A typical food allergy reaction can be the movement, either up or down, of the blood pressure. The patient will not know of this reaction. Insomnia is another symptom which would not necessarily be directly linked to an item in the patient's diet, especially if several foods can bring on the same symptom. Even if the patient avoids one suspect food, another may well produce the same sleepless condition! It can quite quickly become a very confusing picture unless you know how to identify the foods accurately.

So, too, with the person with an underactive thyroid; he may be overweight, but he will not know that it might be specific foods to which he is allergic that are influencing his thyroid so that his metabolic rate chugs along with less efficiency than it might.

The accepted picture of allergies is often the swollen lips upon eating strawberries, or the asthmatic becoming breathless after exposure to an inhalant allergen. The allergies about which this book is written are not so clear-cut, and detective work is required. Indeed, often the eater will feel temporarily better after his allergenic meal, thus throwing him completely off the track (this is 'masked' food allergy, making the eater think the food actually agrees with him).

Again, a reaction will not occur till much later after eating, which can further confuse the poor eater. This delayed reaction means it is highly unlikely any accurate connection will be made between the symptom and any particular food.

If the poor chap was to have bacon and eggs for breakfast in the morning with a couple of cups of coffee, then go to work and have a sandwich or biscuit mid morning with another coffee, then have an early lunch at noon, and a migraine appearing just after his lunch, who would expect the attack to have been caused by the biscuit mid morning, or even the cigarette on the bus on the way to work? It can, and does happen! And it has been happening for hundreds of years and no-one has linked foods to symptoms of ill health in this way until relatively recently.

A What's What of medical ailments can be linked to foods, or chemicals within the foods or in the environment. Common conditions such as arthritis, depression or insomnia are typical of the many complaints which can be shown to be inextricably linked to items in a patient's dietary.

Often, the average G.P. can only prescribe drugs to the sufferer of such symptoms. Undoubtedly these drugs can influence the site of the disorder, but any effect is only temporary. By detecting the offending food items in your diet you will finally be able to find for yourself the actual trigger foods which you must avoid in order to become slim, or remove any stubborn symptoms.

Although the mechanism in food allergy reactions is still unknown, there are theories. One is that many foods contain biologically active chemicals, particularly of the amine group. A good example is the presence of large amounts of tyramine (a commonly occurring amine) in chocolate and cheese. These foods can produce symptoms in susceptible individuals, often a migraine, by a pharmacological action rather like that of a drug.'[11]

It has been shown by the Pottenger Cats experiments (see chapter 11, p. 89) that poor nutrition (cooked meat and heated, pasteurised milk) in the parents can produce kittens with food allergies, whilst another group of cats fed raw meat and unheated milk gave birth to kittens without allergies. So the reason for the widespread obesity that is endemic throughout our modern, 'civilised' societies, is the poor nutrition – the processed, tinned foods – of which the vast majority of us are consumers, creating allergies to foods that interfere with our physiology.

Some people might point to the fact that people in history - like Henry VIII – might have been somewhat on the chubby side and the foods then were not processed or 'interfered' with. I would answer that they were indeed interfered with. They were cooked!

Cooking destroys the enzymes in foods (any heat over 118 deg. F. will render enzymes inactive), so even in those days foods were tampered with. But also, as will be shown later with the Pottenger Cats experiment, allergies can be caused by cooked, deficient diets and can be passed down to your offspring (or at least the susceptibility to allergies can be passed on). Therefore poor Henry's mummy and daddy might well have had diets which were highly cooked, which resulted in food allergies in themselves or in their offspring and consequently these food sensitivities interfered with Henry's metabolism, resulting in his tendency to corpulence. Remember too, that it was the Roman, Lucretius, who recognised that 'What's food for some may be fierce poison for others'.

Food allergies – or sensitivities – are not new. We may only recently have become more aware of them, but as long as it was possible to make a diet deficient – whether by cooking or by any other means – the possibility to create an allergic individual has been there. So the reason for your fatness is food allergy, and the reason for Churchill's fatness was food allergy and the reason for any fat Roman a thousand years ago was food allergy!

As masked food allergy as a phenomenon is showing itself as a cause of a catalogue of health problems, it's no real surprise overweight should be 'just another symptom' to be blamed on the syndrome.

The list of complaints now being shown as directly linked to foods is so diverse that most doctors baulk at the prospect of previously considered 'intractable' complaints being caused by simple foods.

Almost all allergies have been treated with temporary success by the use of the adrenal hormones ACTH and cortisone, which implies that if such treatment is successful, the adrenals must have been malfunctioning in the first place. But as the adrenals are glands themselves and the function of that other gland – the thyroid – can be disrupted, it should be no surprise to consider that these adrenal glands' function are also inhibited by food allergens being ingested. Indeed all the glands, including the pancreas which is involved in blood sugar regulation, are prone to disruption in food allergic responses. Adelle Davis often talked in her books of 'adrenal exhaustion'. Perhaps this book explains why the adrenals should ever become exhausted – by constantly forcing them to malfunction by exposing them to foods that are harmful (allergenic) to these glands!

Hypoglycaemia and Diabetes: the Brother and Sister Conditions

During the 1970s and 1980s hypoglycaemia, meaning low blood sugar, was the buzzword in the United States.

It was the 'fashionable' condition to have. It never quite caught on however, in the U.K. And, because it, like food allergies, could produce almost any symptom, people would blame the condition for their irritability, or bad temper or impatience – even their overweight!

All sorts of high-protein diets were offered as the treatment for the condition, which is the reverse of the same coin with diabetes on the other side. Whilst diabetes is a result of too little of the hormone insulin being produced by the patient's pancreatic gland, hypoglycaemia is the result of the pancreas malfunctioning and over-producing insulin, which lowers blood sugar levels.

Various degrees of success have resulted from differing diets aimed at controlling the condition. All of these diets were of a high animal-protein type. Many people became totally well on these regimens, yet some did not.

There are two types of hypoglycaemia, organic and functional. Organic hypoglycaemia results from malfunctions of the brain, liver, or pancreas, which can be the result of a tumour or diseased organ, whilst functional hypoglycaemia is a group of symptoms often including visual disturbances, sweating, ravenous hunger and nausea, often with trembling, and can fluctuate.

The functional version is often exacerbated by alcohol. The hangover state, especially in the chronic alcoholic, is hypoglycaemia at its most recognisable. Grape juice (not grapefruit juice) drunk last thing at night, or even first thing in the morning, is the best corrector of the alcohol-induced hypoglycaemia.

The fact that some of these high-protein diets would work whilst others would not was because the ones who got well were unwittingly eating a diet free from (their own specific) food allergens. The other hypoglycaemic sufferer, following the same diet to correct the condition, got no better because, unwittingly again, his high-protein menu would contain items to which his pancreas would be allergic.

You will note that I say his *'pancreas would be allergic'*! As Martin L. Budd clearly observes in his book *Low Blood Sugar* 'Medical discoveries are often made by chance rather than by painstaking research and analysis. One open door may lead to others, for much in nature and science is connected.' I have been able to show in this book that the thyroid can be directly influenced by allergenic substances, this then leads us through the next door. The thyroid, like the pancreas, is an endocrine gland. It follows that if one gland can be influenced by incoming food allergens, therefore ALL can be. So it is my firm conviction – and time will bear me out – that hypoglycaemia, whose symptoms would mirror that of the food allergic, is exactly that; the pancreas dysfunctioning as a result of incoming food allergens. *Hypoglycaemia, therefore, is none other than a symptom of food allergy.*

It follows as well that diabetes (hyper-glycaemia), should just be another variation of the same theme and that diabetes will be the result, again, of a malfunctioning pancreatic gland, but this time producing too little insulin as opposed to too much.

As I have shown that the function of the thyroid can be interfered with in allergic responses, so too therefore can the other endocrine glands similarly malfunction because of exposure to offending items in the patient's diet.

But, as not every diabetic pancreas might be responding to allergenic foods, and because of the very real dangers involved with diabetics tampering with their insulin medication, it is absolutely VITAL that, if you are a diabetic, you should not alter your medication – it is essential that you consult your doctor for his advice.

Although the allergenic food theory affecting the pancreas and thus triggering diabetes may not be applicable to ALL diabetics, there will doubtless be very many that it does indeed relate to.

These diabetics will have a faulty pancreas simply because the allergenic foods are interfering with that gland's function and disrupting its blood sugar response. If these diabetics were to remove the food allergens from their diets the gland would recover and in time the condition would become completely controllable without the need for insulin medication. However, I cannot stress enough that any reader who is a diabetic should not apply this approach without professional guidance, as interference with insulin medication can be dangerous.

Candidiasis (or Candida Albicans or Candida)

Like food allergies, like hypoglycaemia, like hypothyroidism, like hyperthyroidism, candida (pronounced can-didda and not can-deeda) is yet another syndrome which had been elevated to the heights of fashion. One wonders what next year's condition will be . . .

I am most certainly NOT suggesting candida is a food allergy symptom (though some may say it's an allergy to yeast-derived organisms), but one thing that candida DOES have in common with the rest, is the fact that all are eminently controllable by diet, as will next year's new condition presently waiting to be labelled; it too, will be controllable by some manipulation of the patient's dietary.

Candida is a result of poor nutrition; of prolonged, long-term consumption of processed, tinned, packaged and denatured foods - foods that are NOT natural to the human body and most certainly not intended by nature to be the desired dietary items by which the body would function at its optimum. The long-term use of antibiotics has also been blamed for the condition. Either way, it is what you put in that hole in your head that has tampered with a naturally-existing organism that would, under proper, *normal*, circumstances, present no cause for concern.

The symptoms common to candida are depression, anxiety, digestive symptoms such as constipation, bloating and heartburn, diarrhoea, fatigue, excessive irritability and an almost permanent sense of impending doom, as well as allergies (!), acne, migraine, cystitis, vaginitis, thrush, menstrual problems and pre-menstrual tension.

We are all, unwittingly perhaps, host to a yeast that lives inside us. This yeast can happily live without causing us any discomfort whatsoever. It is when it spreads out of control that problems can arise. It shouldn't spread, and it wouldn't spread, if we lived (unpopular and boring as it may sound) as nature intended; by consuming foods that are not tampered with and by the avoidance of all drugs (unless of course there is no alternative), which again are unnatural.

Although the drug Nystatin has been touted as *the* answer to the condition, it serves only as a temporary relief. Nystatin is an antifungal antibiotic which can certainly destroy yeast cells on contact. However, if the area of infection of the candida organism is deep within the bowel, then the Nystatin, which can only kill the surface yeasts, will be unable to reach those that may be imbedded deeper into the wall of the intestine.

Whilst it may satisfactorily serve as a palliative, the use of Nystatin does not address the problem of a compromised immune system, which, unless some definite nutritional improvement is applied, will remain weakened.

The use of drugs to combat a condition which can be controlled by a change of diet is much the less desirable option. As with most other drugs, no one is able to say what the long-term cumulative effect of taking unnatural chemical compounds – which drugs are – will be, although the initial side effects of Nystatin are relatively harmless: diarrhoea, nausea and vomiting.

The candida yeast should not spread in the body, but long-term poor nutrition can compromise the integrity of the immune system as well as the efficiency of the mucous membranes which should, under normal conditions, stop that spread occurring.

By the removal of all harmful food substances from the body – food and chemical allergens – and the avoidance of all processed foods, along with the taking up of a completely natural and healthy diet of fruits, vegetables and some nuts or seeds, the health of the individual – as has been shown time and again with such dietary therapies as the Gerson or Nature Cure, will improve to the extent that all the defence systems in the body will function once more and health will be restored – with candida settling down to the harmless yeast that it originally was.

Supplements in Action

Research has indicated that people suffering from allergies are considerably deficient in many nutritional factors, and when these deficiencies are corrected, the allergies disappear. For example, in one such study, children suffering from asthma, hives, or eczema markedly improved when the only change in their diet was the addition of B Complex factors.[12]

Persons with allergies often have abnormally small amounts of vitamin C in their blood.[13] This vitamin acts as a detoxifying agent and has for many years been known to prevent the harmful effects of allergic reactions and anaphylactic shock caused by drugs.

Food allergies cannot occur when foods are completely digested, as simple sugars, amino acids, fatty acids, and glycerin, the products of normal digestion, can never be toxic.[14] It is only when the digestion is in a state of poor health that microscopic particles of undigested, or partially digested food can enter the blood and cause allergic reactions.

Aspirin can make you fat!

In theory, it can. If you are allergic to a prescribed – or otherwise – drug, it may affect your thyroid gland which will result in a slowed metabolism, so to properly carry out the investigation into your allergens you should take this into account, *but you must not stop or reduce any medication you may be on without consulting with your doctor.*

Don't Forget the Chemicals

It may not always be the food itself which is the culprit, but a chemical put in it by the processor or manufacturer. A person may appear to be allergic to a food, let's say an apple, but when the investigation goes further, it may transpire that he is indeed *not* reacting to the apple itself, but to one of the 17 waxes that can be applied during the lifetime of that apple by the distributors or growers in order to make the finished product bright red, shiny, appealing, and more profitable. So the initial thought that he had an allergy to apple might now be changed to awareness that it is a chemical allergy, and he can in fact eat another type of apple.

Not that that would be the end of the story. The chances of someone having an allergy to just one food item are extremely unlikely. Inevitably the poor chap will have other allergies, still waiting to be uncovered.

Foods and the chemicals within them are not the only substances that can cause bodily interference. Alcohol and cigarettes can cause severe responses in susceptible people. And if they are chain-smokers or alcoholics then, with the constant consumption of their drug, their symptoms again will be ever-present and no clear-cut connection will likely be made until proper allergy diagnosis is made. It is estimated, by Clinical Ecologists, that as many as perhaps 70–80 percent of patients who arrive at their doctors' consulting rooms are there for symptoms related to food or chemical allergies. And it's my guess that many of the remainder are there for conditions either attributable to poor nutrition or certainly capable of being improved by some degree of nutritional manipulation.

Allergy or Intolerance?

The substance to which an allergic person can react may be a simple food, or a chemical within that food. It may be something very innocuous, such as a tomato. Or it might well be an airborne allergen such as dust, or tobacco smoke, or fumes from a nearby chemical plant. It could be anything. If it enters your body through your nose, your mouth, or your skin (it might be a soap, the chemicals from which may be absorbed through the skin) then it can be capable of causing an allergic response. Whatever the substance, if you react adversely, and if that substance is not in itself a poison, the fault lies within your own body.

These abnormal reactions to foodstuffs or chemicals etc., are generally referred to as food intolerances,[15] or sensitivities, especially when they are cumulative in effect. These susceptibilities include non-immune disease mechanisms, such as the deficiency of the intestinal enzyme lactase, which produces one form of milk intolerance. The term food 'allergy' is generally reserved for conditions where a specific immune reaction is thought to occur. As allergy means an altered reaction, for the purposes of this book I will refer to all food 'intolerances' as 'allergies', for that is what they truly are.

Breast Feeding May Prevent Allergies

Cow's milk is intended for calves, not for humans. Breast milk is the natural food for the human infant. It has long been suggested that children who are bottle-fed are much more likely to become allergy sufferers than those who are breast fed. As evidenced by the Pottenger Cats' experiment, the health of the mother is vital in determining the degree of health of the offspring, so it is important that the mother feeds well. The mother's need for nutrition is added to by the nutritional demands of the growing foetus within her, and whatever she eats needs to be of a high nutritional quality. The nutritional value of her breast milk, with its immunological implications for the baby, depends on the quality of her diet, not only during gestation, but before conception.

Many studies have been made which show the value of breast milk as an immunological aid to the baby. One in particular[16] showed that the use of formula milks increases the infant's susceptibility to allergy. Ingestion of cow's milk formulas upsets the natural balance of intestinal bacteria and introduces many toxigenic flora, thereby apparently predisposing the infant to allergic tendencies.

In another study[17] 20,061 babies were studied for at least nine months in the United States. Gastrointestinal (GI) and respiratory infections were significantly more frequent in infants fed formula milk. Specifically, deaths from GI infections were sixteen-fold and from respiratory infections over 120-fold more common in cow's milk-fed than breast-fed infants.

Cow's milk is the principal allergen in children and babies. If you have a baby who screams constantly, and is awake half the night yelling blue murder, chances are the child is reacting to something he or she drank – and more than likely it will be cow's milk.

Humans can consume cow's milk without harm, assuming they have the necessary enzymes with which to use the milk efficiently in the first place, and they have been tested and proven not to be allergic to it. In other words, a healthy human should have little problem with cow's milk. But having said that, it must be remembered that in nature no adult animal drinks milk of any kind. That tells me that it might be no bad thing to forego milk as a drink, particularly pasteurised and especially if your family has displayed an allergic history. And don't panic over the possible lack of protein which milk supplies: the protein myth is another one which I dispel in this book. However, wherever man has taken milk, in primitive, healthy peoples, their milk has been raw and unpasteurised. Our ordinary bottled cow's milk is not raw and it is heated during pasteurisation, therefore it is deficient.

Cow's milk can be a highly allergic food not only to babies but to adults too. And it can remain an unrecognised source of health problems for a person's entire lifespan. However, with this book you will be able to ascertain all your allergic foods and drinks, and as well as losing all your surplus fat, perhaps other complaints which you have learned to live with will clear up.

The 'Target Organs'

It is still little understood why one person, when reacting to an allergen, will produce symptoms in one part of the body, time and again, whilst another person, consuming the same food, or inhaling the same airborne pollutant, and who is also an allergy sufferer, will produce symptoms in an entirely different part of the body. The 'target organ' in each of the individuals will be different but that same target organ will be the reacting site every time an allergen is ingested.

Whilst patient A might get depression every time he consumes a cream cake, patient B might get a rash on his legs when he eats the very same substance. The target areas are at opposite ends of the body, but it appears each person has his own inherited weak spot or the weakness has been 'randomly' created by previous poor diet adversely affecting that area.

Allergic reactions can appear in almost any part of the body and they occur internally as well as externally. The itching on the skin of the arm might be very obvious and evident to the sufferer, but there can be more subtle, INTERNAL reactions of which you will know nothing. The food allergy influence on the thyroid gland and its metabolic implications is one superb overlooked example.

Nevertheless, the reason for different target organs being 'attacked' in allergic reactions in different individuals is still a mystery, but an accepted phenomenon. Besides the commonly accepted probability of an inherited weakness it may be that the person has been born with a *susceptibility* to arthritis say, but would never have developed the full-blown condition, IF his diet from birth had been a completely natural one and free from adulterants. But, given the state of our nutrition today, it may also be that the constant feeding of nutritionally-deficient foodstuffs since birth has slowly and surely further weakened what was already a potential weakspot in the first place. And that susceptibility, that weakness, latent though it may have been initially, has now become a full-blown, constantly-reacting symptom of distress.

The Immune System

An explanation as to why some people can have many allergies yet others remain free from the condition is explained later in this book, but the answer to the question as to why many people fall prey to symptoms such as the common cold whilst others manage to comfortably dodge the coughing and sniffling that goes with the territory, is often laid at the door of our fascinating immune system.

Why some people suffer regular infections whilst others escape, depends on a highly complex network of infection-fighting activities. One type depends on our white blood cells, which remove external particles, including viruses, bacteria, plant and animal material. Another type of activity depends on circulating proteins, known as humoral antibodies or immunoglobulins, which react and pair with specific foreign substances (antigens), neutralising them. In addition, other important protective proteins (such as properdin, complement, interferon) are classified as non-specific factors which help to maintain the level of immune response. Finally, the skin and mucous membranes contribute to our good health by protecting us against the entry of bacterial and viral invaders.[18]

It has been shown that there is an intimate relationship between nutritional deficiencies and infection and indeed, allergies.[19,20] Elderly people are often susceptible to infection and research into the effects of nutritional supplementation for just eight weeks on the nutrition and immunocompetence of elderly persons showed that nutritional support increased immune responses.[21]

A diet deficient in vitamins B1, B2, folic acid, biotin, or niacin inhibits the production of antibodies and white blood cells, though less severely than when pantothenic acid (Vit B5) or Vitamin B6 is limited.[22,23,24]

The immune system is the no. 1 suspect in degenerative disease and in premature ageing.[25] It is really split into two interdependent parts – the thymus with its T-lymphocytes or T-cells, which is the main system of cellular immunity, and the B-lymphocytes or B-cells which protect us from most viral and bacterial infections.

Adelle Davis, in her book *Lets Get Well* states: 'During the past two decades, Dr. Fred R. Klenner, of Reidsville, North Carolina, has used massive quantities of Vitamin C in treating successfully patients of all ages suffering from such serious illnesses as encephalitis, meningitis, poliomyelitis, viral pneumonia, tetanus, or lockjaw, and many other infections. Usually these patients had an extremely high fever, were unconscious, and many had been given up earlier by physicians who believed them to be beyond help: some appeared to be dying, and in one case rigor mortis had actually set in! To extremely ill patients Dr. Klenner gave the vitamin by injection in amounts ranging from 2 to 4 grams (2,000 to 4,000 milli-grams) approximately every two to four hours around the clock, the amount and number of injections depending on the progress of each individual. Sometimes he gave antibiotics or other medications in addition to vitamin C, although these drugs had usually been given by other physicians before the patients had become so desper-ately ill. An amazing number of these persons regained consciousness quickly, were able to drink juices within a few hours, took further vitamin C by mouth, and were discharged from hospital in three or four days.'

Practically any nutrient deficiency can affect the efficient working of the immune system, so every attempt should be made to maximise the quality of your dietary. Your diet should be unrefined – as natural as possible – as uncooked as possible, and of course, free from all aller-genic substances, in order to give the reacting organs a rest so that they may heal.

THREE

What Happens When We Eat Our Food

The food on the table in front of you may be elaborately arranged. It may be supremely colourful and exotic, superbly attractive to the eye. And that is all good and well. There may be a coloured little umbrella cheekily protruding over the top of the cocktail glass. The flickering, romantic candlelight adds to the appeal of the occasion. It all whets the appetite. Every effort is made by the lady of the house (or the man!) to make the meal an adventure; a work of art even. And we are the only animals on earth with this luxury. For that is what it is.

The poor tiger has no such frills. His meal stalks through the jungle on four dirty feet and is inevitably totally covered in manky hair. But the result is the same. The meals should supply nutrition to the eater. The better the nutrition, the healthier the body.

The tiger may be without the knife and fork, the romantic candlelight, and the coloured arrangement of the meal on the pine table but he will unquestionably be better nourished than the vast majority of humans on earth.

The tiger's meal will be as nature intended: live, uncooked, unrefined, un-tampered-with; whilst our exotic offering on the dining room table may well be many days, or even weeks, old; grown from poor soil; interfered with by food processing; and heavily cooked into the bargain.

Repeat such a nutritional abomination three times a day, 365 days a year, and times it by forty and we have almost 44,000 meals by the time we get to middle age. There is no way in the world that so much food can go through a person without it having an effect on him. And it further stands to reason that if these 44,000 meals were complete in their nutritional content (enzymes and nutrients) then the eater would have better health than if his 44,000 meals consisted of 44,000 plates of refined and processed foods, deficient in every nutrient known (and unknown), to man. And do not think that *you* do not eat such deficient foods, because it is almost certain that if you shop for your foods at an everyday super-market or grocers, you will be putting inside yourself meals of a deficient and denatured quality. And if you are overweight, or have symptoms of illhealth, look at your plate for the answer, because that is where it will most certainly lie!

But what happens to the food we eat? How does the body utilise all that food, and for what purpose?

The mere sight of food, whether it be the colourful offering on the dining table, or the manky hyena stumbling through the undergrowth, establishes the flow of saliva. The chewing of the food activates not only more saliva but also a chemical reflex which is conveyed to the stomach, where gastric juices prepare for the oncoming traffic.

How science came to study the activity in the stomach is an interesting story. In 1822, 18-year-old Alex St. Martin[26] was accidentally shot in the chest by a musket, from a range of only three feet. The appalling wound was treated by pushing the lungs and stomach back, and attempting to close the aperture with stitches. Against all expectation, he survived. A week later he was eating as normal, except that most of what he ate came out through the remaining hole in his abdomen. In spite of this, he lived on, and the 'window' in his stomach was the first insight into the workings of the digestive system. Through it, the actual process of digestion could be seen, and samples of digestive fluids could be taken.

The chewed-up food is swallowed and passes down the oesophagus (the gullet) by a wormlike movement called peristalsis, which squeezes the food down the 23 cm journey to the stomach. This wave of constriction is usually initiated by the actual swallowing of food, and, in the words of the great Naturopath, James C. Thomson, of the Kingston Clinic[27]: 'It is normal for naturally-living animals to produce a bowel movement soon after eating. Peristalsis begins at the back of the mouth; the action of swallowing causes the constricting wave to pass down the gullet, carrying the food with it. Although the far end of the stomach is temporarily closed, the wave continues beyond it and passes through the whole length of the gut. The first waves of a series are usually much stronger than succeeding ones, and 'strip' the intestines downward, towards the rectum. This leaves the upper reaches of the digestive tract free from stale debris, and thus able to concentrate upon the newly-arriving food.'

Back to the action in the stomach. There, digestive juices, which are secreted from the abdominal walls, and enzymes, churn and mix the food until it has the consistency of a thick liquid, called chyme. If, however, the eater has digestive problems then the juices may be insufficient to break down the foods and this can result in some of the foodstuffs travelling the entire length of the alimentary canal and coming out the other end almost entirely unaltered!

This chyme will now enter a tubelike structure called the duodenum, which carries it to the small intestine. Before it does this, more digestive juices and enzymes which come from the nearby pancreas and gallbladder, mix with the chyme to reduce it even further. These juices and enzymes help to reduce the fats, proteins, and carbohydrates in preparation for the rest of the journey. The carbohydrates are reduced to simple sugars called glucose, galactose, and fructose, whilst the fats are reduced to minute droplets known as micelles. Protein is broken down into amino acids. During the journey through the small intestine, the various nutrients find affinity with different sections, where they are absorbed into the bloodstream. Whatever is not needed by the body for nutrition will continue until it is eliminated through the anus as faeces. Meanwhile, the foods which have managed to leave the small intestine will all meet up again in the tiny blood capillaries and lymph vessels and continue on their travel.

The amino acids and sugars travel along the portal vein which connects to the liver. The pumping of the heart keeps the bloodstream moving and the nutrients are swiftly moved along on their journey. The blood capillaries are minute vessels that can be likened to the tributaries of a river, and through them the microscopic food particles (because that is what they have been reduced to by now) travel on their way to the liver, via the portal vein.

The liver is the supreme gland of the body, and sits on the right side under the rib cage. It is one of the largest organs of the body and is vital to life. Drinking alcohol and even eating refined junk foods over a long time can damage the liver. But it is so versatile that up to half of this amazing organ can be damaged and, given the right nutrition, it is capable of regenerating itself to its former glory!

We can live without arms, legs, even one lung or one kidney, but without the liver we would die.

The liver can destroy harmful substances which might enter it from the central bloodstream (from the lungs and heart) or from the portal bloodstream (from the intestines). Hormones carrying information about the requirements of different parts of the body are released into the liver from the bloodstream and simple sugars in the form of glucose, and amino acids, are deployed according to the requirements.

Each one of us is composed of about 100 trillion tiny cells. They join together to form bones, muscles, fat, skin and other tissues and organs. These cells need constantly to be nourished, and the food we eat is the only nourishment they get.

The minute food particles that have now been reduced so far that they would only be visible under a microscope are finally delivered to the cells as nourishment by the microscopic blood capillaries.

The Calorie Myth

Many slimming experts still insist that control of obesity is simply a case of taking in less calories than you would expel in energy, and therefore, if you reduce your calorific intake, you will lose weight. Yet many fat people eat very little and still they cannot lose weight!

These experts are not taking into account a possibly inefficient metabolism.

The calorie fallacy has been exploded by such pioneers in diet as Mackarness, Blake Donaldson, Dr. Atkins, etc. All of them would give patients diets of high fat, low or zero-carbohydrate, and therefore very high-calorie composition, sometimes in excess of 3,000 calories per day. And they lost weight beautifully! Eskimos, too, consume diets very high in calories, and although they may appear tubby, this is an illusion, due to the swathing of numerous layers of warm clothing. They have fine builds and it is only a racial feature which makes their faces appear roundish. Dr. V. E. Levine of Omaha, Nebraska, examined 3,000 primitive Eskimos during 3 trips to the Arctic and found only one overweight person!.[28] It all comes down to the efficiency of your thyroid gland and so, your metabolism.

If calories were the only factor involved in weight control then people who can eat anything and still not put on weight would simply not exist. Their mere presence in our society throws the whole calorie issue out of the window. If Tom can eat 3,000 calories a day and not put on weight, whilst Dick eats 3,000 calories a day but the poor fellow balloons, then it stands to reason that the calorie factor *cannot* be the only issue

Why then does the calorie-controlled diet, popular with doctors and slimming clubs, *appear* to work? I use the word 'appear' because many people on low calorie diets still cannot lose weight, whilst others – who are iron-willed enough to adhere to them – can reduce, but often with great difficulty.

I hope herein to give the correct explanation for the popular calorie-counting 'success'.

If you eat a food which causes an allergic response in your thyroid gland's function, the degree of dysfunction in this cumulative allergy will depend on the quantity of the harmful substance eaten. Therefore if you eat a large – and continuous – amount of such a food then the metabolism will slow down greatly, never able to match the intake of foodstuffs, resulting in overweight. The more allergenic foods you eat, the greater the adverse affect on your thyroid gland.

A smaller amount of allergenic food creates less dysfunction, and for a shorter duration, than a consistent bombardment of large amounts of the offending foodstuffs.

Therefore, a low calorie diet, with its decreased quantity of food will, unwittingly, reduce the thyroid gland's exposure to the harmful, allergenic foodstuffs, which in turn lessens the degree of malfunction in the gland and so the eater can show signs of near-normal metabolism!

However, as the number of failures on such a regimen will testify, low-calorie living is not easy to adhere to. Primitive peoples, such as the Hunzakuts, and indeed, the Eskimos, are extremely healthy – and slim – yet eat considerably larger quantities of foods than the often-quoted under-1,000 calories a day given by slimming clubs.

So, in low-calorie-controlled-diets, it is not simply the reduction in calories which can sometimes reduce the person's weight, but the avoidance of, or great reduction in, the thyroid-affecting foodstuffs in that reduced diet.

There is a basic principle behind the calorie approach that would make sense in a perfect world. But our overweight people do not have perfect metabolisms – or they wouldn't be overweight in the first place!

The calorie principle does not apply to the mass of people who are overweight because of a disturbed metabolism. If you were to eat nothing at all, then your body's metabolism would still be working whilst nothing was incoming, so yes, whilst fasting you would most cer-

tainly lose weight. But in the case of the vast majority of
people who have a less-than-efficient thyroid function and
are thus overweight, the low-calorie approach will only
work with extremely low calorie menus (near to fasting).
It is almost impossible to adhere to this approach for any
length of time, and it is certainly unnatural.

As some of the cases elsewhere in this book testify,
there are patients who had unlimited access to sugar –
white, deadly, and frighteningly-high calorie sugar – and
who continued to lose weight simply because they were
not allergic to it, therefore it was not causing their thyroid
to malfunction. Yet the calorific value of sugar, as we
all might know, is about 400 calories in a small 3oz
helping!

There are people who cannot lose any weight whatsoever on even a 500 calorie diet![29] This too, highlights the
almost certain possibility that such people, although on
very low calorific diets, are acutely allergic to the contents
of their meagre fare, and they might well lose weight on a
very much *higher* calorie diet IF it were composed of foods
that did not adversely affect their metabolic glands.

FOUR

How to Test for Food Allergies at Home

One of the most accurate methods of testing for food and chemical allergies is by the monitoring of your pulse. Hospital skin tests for food allergies have been shown to be notoriously unreliable indicators.

Monitoring your pulse and watching for a speeding up or slowing down after eating, can be an extremely accurate guide to identifying culprit foods or drinks within your diet.

Caution

If you are prone to asthma or epilepsy, and as food allergies can produce such symptoms, it is essential that this programme of testing only be followed under strict medical supervision.

Your pulse should be at its lowest reading first thing in the morning, before you get out of bed. However, if you indulged in a heavy meal the night before, full of allergenic foods, your morning's pulse reading might still be affected by such foods and this is a phenomenon that you will have to be aware of during testing.

Your aim is to arrive at your normal lowest pulse. This may take a few days to achieve as you remove, one by one, allergenic foods from your diet, but once your meals are free from foods that affect you, only *then* should your morning reading show your true, minimum pulse rate.

If your morning pulse rate is not the lowest reading of the day, suspect something in your bedroom or environment (perhaps the pilot light of the gas fire, a new carpet, or even the bedding) as possibly influencing your pulse. Be aware also that seemingly innocuous items like fresh newsprint, soap, or even toothpaste can have a bearing on your pulse. If they do, you're allergic to them.

Once your lowest pulse rate is established, there are certain features of food/chemical allergies that can be accurately applied and used as a guide to assess your progress. These are:

(1) From your lowest pulse reading of the day to your highest should not exceed 16 beats – assuming freedom from illness, strenuous exercise, or sunburn.
(2) Your pulse reading should differ little when sitting or standing; if it does it indicates existing allergic tension.
(3) Psychological influences will have no bearing on the pulse rate of a healthy individual.
(4) A rested pulse reading above 84 indicates allergy.

The textbook 'average' pulse is 72, but everybody has their own individual normal rate and you will be able to identify your normal, healthy, pulse reading as your food testing progresses and allergenic foods are removed from your diet.

How To Take Your Pulse

Turn your left hand over, so that it is palm up. Take the first two fingers of your right hand and place them on the centre of your left wrist about an inch down from where the hand joins the wrist. Now move the fingers to halfway between where your fingers have just been, and the outer (left) edge of the wrist. There is no need for heavy pressure; a light pressure will let you now feel the pulse. The more you practise taking the pulse the easier it will be to find it. You will soon become as adept at taking it as any doctor!

For food allergy testing purposes it is important that you take the count for a full 60 seconds; not for 30 seconds then multiplying by 2 as nurses do. Because a mere few beats can mean the difference between safe or culprit food, and as multiplying by four may well arrive at a less-than-accurate reading, the full minute's count is essential.

To get an accurate full minute's reading, start the count after the second hand leaves the 12 and finish the count when the second hand arrives back and lands on the 12.

On the day you decide to start your food tests, take your pulse before you get out of bed. This reading will probably get lower as the days progress and as you discover and remove allergenic foods from your diet. It is essential that you keep a food diary, writing down everything you eat and drink and at what time, along with your pulse readings.

Make three columns in your diary with these headings;-

(1) Safe Foods (2) Forbidden Foods (3) Under Suspicion

Test your meals by taking your pulse just before eating, then taking it again three more times after the meal, each half an hour apart. Write down the pulse readings. If your pulse accelerates or slows down by five or more beats after eating, then that food must go in the forbidden column. Your pulse will not be affected by ordinary physical activity so it is not essential to sit still like a dummy for the entire 90 minutes awaiting the pulse readings! However, for the three readings during testing it is always best to sit down for a few minutes prior to taking the pulse so as to ensure an unconfusing picture.

After a few days some sort of pattern will emerge and you will be able to spot the meals which influenced your pulse. However, you may not know which of the ingredients within that meal caused the pulse to be affected.

The reason for testing entire meals for a few days is to get you into the way of testing and at the same time hopefully give you a recognisable pattern of pulse-influencing mealtimes which will serve to prove to you that you indeed have food allergies!

You can now choose your day in which to isolate and test individual foods. That day should start, as usual, with your first pulse-taking of the day, in bed.

The second pulse reading will be seated, just before your first test meal. You should eat an average-sized portion of a regularly consumed food; say, potatoes. Do not add anything such as butter or pepper; you are testing only the actual food.

After eating the food, take your pulse again 30 minutes later, then a further 30 minutes later, and the final reading a further 30 minutes on. That is:

(i)   Take your pulse before the meal, then
(ii)   30 minutes after eating
(iii) 60 minutes after eating
(iv)   90 minutes after eating

If your pulse moves – up or down – 5 or more beats from the pre-meal reading, allergy is indicated. If you get any symptoms – say headache, or dizziness – even without a pulse change, this can still be indicative of food allergy and that particular food should go in the 'Under Suspicion' columnn, to be tested again at a later date to see if these symptoms appear again. This re-testing of foods that may not influence the pulse but may bring on symptoms should only be carried out *five days* after the first test.

If, after the 90 minutes have passed, your pulse has not changed and no symptoms have occurred, that food can be put in the 'Safe' column and you may start your next food test immediately. However, if your pulse does change or if any symptoms should appear, you must wait until both your pulse returns to the pre-test reading and the symptoms have worn off before starting your next food test.

A typical pulse diary – when testing foods – would look something like this:

| | | | Pulse Readings | | |
Time	Food	Before Food	After 30 mins	After 60 mins	After 90 mins
12 noon	Grapes	68	68	68	68
1.30 pm	Bananas	68	75	83	74

(On the above test, grapes – if you did not get any symptoms during the testing – are safe. But the bananas caused the pulse to jump more than 5 beats (it jumped 15 at its highest) so would definitely go in the Forbidden column, whether or not you get any symptoms).

You would wait until your pulse returns to 68 after the banana test – and any symptoms have gone – before proceeding with the next food test.

The symptoms that may occur might be as innocent as belching, or a feeling of bloated stomach, or wind, or a vague headache – indeed any odd feeling may occur. If you get any of these, then put that food in the Under Suspicion column, and write beside it 'belching' – or whatever symptoms you had, along with the date, so that you will remember when to re-test. Then test again five days later, and if the same symptoms occur, put that food in the Forbidden column.

You will continue testing in the above fashion until you identify all your food allergens.

The multiple food test

Not for the faint-hearted, but it certainly can be a short cut! You can, instead of laboriously testing one food every 90 minutes, try a four or five-food test. Ideally these should be foods which are unlikely to prove allergenic (say, vegetables – although this is not always the case). You would eat the five portions at the one sitting, applying the same principles as before – taking the pulse before eating and then every 30 minutes after until 90 minutes had expired. If no symptoms or pulse change, then these four or five foods would be considered safe. However, if it transpires that the combined foods do in fact affect your pulse, then you are almost back to square 1 as you will have to re-test every single one of these foods at a later date (minimum five days later). So, although it can be a short cut if no reaction occurs, it can set you back a bit if the meal proves allergenic. It is perhaps a technique best left until you are well into the testing, when you have a large list of safe foods and any setback won't be too bothersome.

As you remove the offending foods from your diet, your estimate of your lowest morning reading will change, until you arrive at your true minimal pulse reading. When this is reached you must remember that, as long as your diet is free from allergenic foods, and you do not have an illness, your pulse range during the day should not exceed 16 beats above your morning's reading. It is normal for the healthy pulse to increase during the day but if it increases above 16 beats over your morning reading, you have been exposed to an allergen; whether food, drink, or inhalant.

When testing liquids such as tea, coffee, milk, vegetable juices or even tap water, there is a quicker method which you can apply. Again, take your pulse before the test. Then swirl the liquid round your mouth and hold it under your tongue with your head held slightly tilted back and retain it there for one full minute, then swallow.

You then only need to take your pulse (for the usual full minute's reading) at 15 minute intervals three times. That is;

(i)   Take your pulse before the drink, then
(ii)   15 minutes after drinking
(iii) 30 minutes after drinking
(iv)   45 minutes after drinking

You may consider that testing tap water is being over-cautious, but it is not common knowledge that tap water can have small amounts of pesticides in it as well as other adulterants, and these can indeed influence the pulse.

You should remember that, as your testing progresses and your normal diet is split into safe and unsafe foods, so then will the need for testing reduce as you gather more and more information about the way in which your commonly-eaten foods affect you as an individual. The most testing always takes place at the beginning and diminishes as you progress through your diet until you are satisfied that you have covered all the foods that you would regularly be exposed to. You will notice, as the testing progresses and you are therefore eating less foods which will be adversely influencing the function of your thyroid gland, your weight will start to drop off. It will all have been so worth it!

Blood Tests for Food Allergies

For those of you who may find the above too time-consuming, there is a reputable nutritional laboratory who can offer blood tests for food allergies. There is a huge advantage in this if you can afford it (cost for approximately 70 foods to be tested from the one blood sample is apparently £90-odd at time of going to print but compared to others – who can charge £135, it can represent good value and it is certainly a short cut!). They are:

The York Nutritional Laboratory
Dept. ABAP
Tudor House
Lysander Close
Clifton Moor
York   Telephone 0990 100812

Loose, sagging skin as a result of large weight loss

With large weight losses, this is a phenomenon many readers will be aware of, and is the result of reducing diets which pay little heed to the actual QUALITY of the nutrition supplied, or whether the foods in that diet were allergenic to that particular individual, thus adversely affecting the biochemical-physiological internal environment. With the taking-up of a diet largely composed of natural, unprocessed foods, the skin will in time restore itself to its natural tautness.

Many people have resorted to surgery in order to correct the problem when mere attention to the actual QUALITY of their nutrition would have achieved the desired effect.

PHANTOM REACTIONS AND THE DIETER'S 'PLATEAU

People who are overweight are the result of a simple equation, namely: food goes in but not all of it comes out!

That crude observation may be deceptively simplistic, but it is a fact. It has to be accepted that it is not the air that we breathe that makes us swell and shows up on the scales as extra pounds or stones in weight − it is the food that we have consumed that is incompletely 'burned' by our much-slowed-down, faulty metabolism, and incompletely eliminated. Effectively these metabolic wastes − these food residues − are retained within the system.

The normal body has the ability to store away nutritive materials that are put away in the form of fat, glycogen, bone marrow, muscle juices, lacteal fluids, vitamins and minerals.

But besides this normal, and natural, famine-combatting facility that Nature has thoughtfully provided man, someone with a disordered metabolism and probably too, disturbed digestive capabilities, will retain other metabolic wastes.

The metabolism in the allergic person who gains weight easily is slowed down to the extent that it cannot properly cope with even a 'normal' amount of incoming food and has no option other than to 'store' it.

Many of you who have lost weight on other diets − most likely the calorie-restricted variety − will have at some time hit the famous dieter's 'Plateau'; a time when, even although you are faithfully adhering to your diet, the weight loss comes to a halt. It is a frustrating experience for which there seems no logical explanation.

Experts around the world have tried in vain to successfully explain this demoralising phenomenon: I will now give you the REAL explanation.

When you do lose weight – by whatever means – that extra, stored weight, naturally enough leaves your body. This extra weight you will remember, is to all intents and purposes the residue of previously eaten foods – the foods that went in, but did not come out.

When these wastes eventually dissolve, in preparation for final elimination from your body, they re-enter the bloodstream and circulate once more round your system.

As some of these stored microscopic food residues will almost certainly have been foods to which you would have been allergic, that re-circulating of these previously-eaten foods, if sufficiently copious in quantity, can create a brand new allergic reaction whilst in your bloodstream, awaiting elimination!

When this happens, your thyroid gland will once more be adversely affected and your metabolism will grind to a halt. The weight loss temporarily stops and you have arrived at the notorious 'Plateau'!

The same phenomenon applies if you would normally experience food allergic symptoms: during the re-circulating of old food residues, again, it will be as if you have just eaten that allergenic food and your headache, or your depression, or whatever symptom you normally experience with food allergies, will return. And the tantalising thing is that you may well blame it on an actual food eaten an hour or so ago, when in fact, that food was blameless and the headache is being caused by a food eaten three months previously!

THIS IS A 'PHANTOM REACTION'

As your weight returns to normal and the stored wastes in your body become less and less, these 'phantom' reactions will reduce in number and your true allergic picture will become easier to decipher. However, it is an occurrence of which few food allergy therapists are aware and it must be taken into account when any unexplained recurrence of symptoms appears.

Available Tests for Food Allergies

There are several tests available commercially for food and chemical allergies. They are:

RAST (Radioallogeosorbent test) which is a blood test that measures the IgE levels in response to a given allergen. However, there are too many imponderables that need to be taken into account which makes it unreliable, with false negatives commonplace.

Cytotoxic Test Another blood test. This one extracts the white cells and platelets, mixes them with serum and sterile water and puts them in contact with the suspect substances. Its accuracy extends to around 80 percent and it is an encouragingly quick route to identifying a host of possible substances and an excellent base from which to further expand your own investigations.

Vega Tests This is an electrical testing device which is a version of the Wheatstone bridge. It tests the electrical response of the body, through probes pressed on the fingertips, to substances placed within the circuit. As the patient can actually see the machine's responses, it has a positive motivatory influence to stay on a given diet. But, even with a skilled practitioner, the results are approximately 75 percent accurate.

Patch Testing Quantities of suspected substances are put under patches which are taped to the skin for a number of hours. A reddening of the skin (barring a sensitivity to the pad or tape itself) would suggest a sensitivity to that substance. But this testing is often unreliable, due to negative responses having occurred on substances known to be allergenic.

Applied Kinesiology A relatively 'unscientific' method wherein the practitioner can diagnose a sensitivity to a substance even if the patient only happens to be holding a glass bottle containing the substance, by checking the resistance of certain muscles. From my own experience of it, it is not without merit, with considerable potential if in the hands of a skilled practitioner.

The slower but generally more effective tests are the direct challenge tests with the actual food, either in conjunction with, or without, the added diagnostic aid of pulse testing.

Sublingual Tests/Pulse test A direct challenge test, with a liquid extract of the food placed under the tongue for a swift delivery to the bloodstream. The pulse is monitored at the same time. Some practitioners doubt the pulse technique's validity and state that there can be several false positives and false negatives. In other words the pulse may rise but there is no reaction from the patient (false positive) or there is a false negative (pulse doesn't move but reaction occurs). There can be reasons for these: a pulse rise with no obvious symptom response only means that the patient is *unaware* of any reaction. As stated before, some physiological reactions, such as a drop in blood pressure, or some adverse influence on the thyroid or other glands, may be taking place unbeknown to the patient. But the mere fact that the food has made the pulse rise is in *itself* a reaction, because if it rises say 7 beats without any obvious recurrence of symptoms, that means that the practitioner is ignoring a food substance which is capable of increasing the massively powerful heartbeats. Although seven beats per minute may not seem much, *seventy* beats every ten minutes is surely a significant reaction in itself.

A false NEGATIVE, whereby no pulse change is recorded but there is a reaction when later the food is taken, can be because certain foodstuffs are not readily absorbed into the bloodstream (as in cereal grains for example) but when cooked and eaten, a true reaction can take place. Therefore, given the proper interpretation

of the testing, sublingual challenging in conjunction with
pulse taking, can be one of the most effective methods
of testing for food/chemical allergens, next to the actual
swallowing of the foods themselves.

FIVE

Withdrawal Symptoms

This is the nitty gritty! This is the reason why there are so many intelligent, fat people about: so many intelligent smokers, alcoholics and drug addicts. Intelligence can actually be a hindrance, as it endows the sufferer – for that is what he is – with a false sense of being in control. Once an addict (whether to food or cigarettes or drugs) removes the addictive substance from his regular consumption, severe withdrawal symptoms can arise. Even if you use my approach to identify your allergenic foods, it may well be that you have become addicted to some of them, in which case an element of willpower will need to be applied.

The structure behind the withdrawal phenomenon has yet to be explained fully by physiologists, but essentially the same mechanism is involved no matter whether we are coming off cigarettes, coffee, chocolate, alcohol, favourite foods, or drugs.

Of course, the degree of severity of the symptoms will vary, all the way from hardly any symptoms at all, to wishing you had never been born!

These withdrawal symptoms can show up as weepiness; emotional instability; fatigue; sleepiness and all the emotions from plain irritability to out-and-out rage!

The subtle intricacies of the addiction process are almost beyond comprehension, unless you have personally witnessed the cunning 'internal' manipulation – seemingly against your will – that takes place. The same process applies to all addictions, no matter the substance.

For ease of explanation I will talk about cigarettes for the moment, but substitute your own favourite food or drink for the word cigarette, as the information applies equally to all.

The 'Oh, I'll just have this one more cigarette, and I promise myself I will *definitely*, most *definitely* stop tommorrow' syndrome is one that the majority of smokers have experienced. It is a dismissal of the addiction. It is attempting to say that 'I' am in control and not the cigarette. In other words *I* will stop when I am good and ready and today I am not, but tommorrow I will be!

Such is the blinding nature of addiction. It really is like you against them, your brain against the will of another brain. There does indeed seem to be a little angel on one shoulder telling you what you know in your heart of hearts you should do, and a little devil on the other shoulder telling you quite emphatically that having another fag is no problem whatsoever, and in fact it would be quite a good idea, and besides, you know damn fine you can stop it whenever you want to!

That is the tremendously clever, extremely subtle conflict that every person with an addiction goes through, whether he has analysed it or not.

Before you started smoking, it would have seemed incomprehensible if someone were to have told you that by repeated smoking of cigarettes there would be created a most powerful craving for that substance within your body. You might have known other people who succumbed to such an addiction, but deep down you would have ignored the possibility of such overpoweringly compulsive behaviour happening within your own body. But it always happens.

It may start off as one cigarette a day; and you may start off with every intention in the world not to let it increase; but it will nearly always slowly creep up until you may well be on forty or so a day.

But the fact that at one time you could live without cigarettes shows that you weren't BORN with this particular addiction. The particular affinity of your brain for that substance has been acquired. And, equally, like millions of other people who used to smoke but have now given up, or drank alcohol and have now abandoned it for a purer life, you can arrive back at that state in which you do not crave these substances. But it needs work. The addiction has to be fought.

The intensity of your withdrawal symptoms depends on the severity of the addiction – and the substance. For example, although it is not necessary to 'wean' yourself off your addictive foods (although you may choose to do so!), it is essential in powerful addictions such as to drugs or alcohol that a weaning-off process is undergone, and this MUST be under the supervision of your doctor.

Most smokers know how difficult it can be trying to give it up. It can be horrendous. But not impossible! As an ex-smoker too, I know it can be beaten. As long as the desire to stop smoking, or to stop any addiction, is there, then if you follow the advice in this book, the craving *will* be beaten!

Food addiction – and we are talking about foods that, if you crave them then there is an excellent chance of your being allergic to them – can be as powerful in the craving department as cigarettes.

The cravings behind the allergic reaction have a real physical trigger. And that trigger is a neurotransmitter called serotonin.

Food allergics often, once they eat something they are allergic to, go on a binge of that very food, or other foods to which they are allergic (which they crave). The appetite can become almost uncontrollable and can explain the bingeing behaviour of all the fat people in our Westernised societies. The reason why food allergic individuals should, once they have consumed a food allergen, go on an 'allergic binge' of the very foods that they are reacting to can perhaps be at least partly explained by one study into the levels of serotonin in the blood.

The study showed that during a migraine reaction (which will almost certainly have been caused by a food)[30] there is a drop in the blood level of serotonin.

Pharmacological, biochemical and behavioural evidence has accumulated in the last two decades suggesting that brain serotonin has an inhibitory influence on eating behaviour both in animals and in humans.[31] Reported studies in favour of a possible role played by the serotoninergic system in the explanation of anorexia present in different diseases further support this idea.[32,33]

As the level of serotonin plays an important part in hunger; and given that the serotonin levels drop during a migraine attack, and as migraine is an allergic reaction, it is not unreasonable to think that in ALL food allergic reactions, the blood levels of this neurotransmitter will be affected. The uncontrollable appetite which follows from this is a state similar to the withdrawal symptoms when the allergic person craves his food. The allergenic food will be interfering not only with other physiological processes within the body, but also with the serotonin level, and in the withdrawal from the food, as with all drug withdrawal conditions, there is often a (temporary) increase in the severity of the body's malfunctioning.

This will also account for the fat person's age-old dilemma (remember serotonin, although recently discovered, was in Henry VIII's blood too, all these years ago!): when he eats something 'fattening' he can't stop. As I am saying the fat man's obesity is due to food allergy, then, as he ingests the foods to which he is allergic, this triggers the drop in blood serotonin, which in turn creates the appetite (or craving) which can appear almost uncontrollable.

That is why there are so many fat people who know what they *should* do, but cannot do it. There is a real biochemical conflict going on; your own logic against the neurotransmitter serotonin! It is not a mere 'whim' that you may want more of that pie you've just eaten, and to which you are allergic. It is a real physiological cry for help from your serotonin!

This phenomenon appears constantly in withdrawals from the addictive substance. And if the person tries to 'fight' the desire, he will suffer great unease, even depression. If he loses the battle inside his head with himself, and decides to give into and indeed HAVE that slice of gateau or that other pie, the depression will miraculously lift, even before he has his first bite! The mere *decision*, which no onlooker will know he arrived at, the mere knowledge that within the next half hour or so he is going to have his beloved gateau, can suddenly turn his gloom around into utter and true joy! His life will suddenly be rosy! Spring will have sprung! Life will be worth living again!

That is what happens if you give in to the depression of withdrawal, and go back to the substance that you are addicted to. Indeed that is a method of telling if you ARE addicted to something. If you decide to give it up, feel downcast, and realise that, if you take it once again, life will be so much better, even although temporarily, then that, my friend, is the mechanism of addiction in its simplest, but commonest, form!

The subtleties are so complex in withdrawals. It appears that every trick, every deception that can be played by *another* brain is actively involved in trying to get you to succumb to your own brain's powerful and incessant demand for the substance.

When you stop taking the substance you are addicted to, you will have withdrawls (or if you are not severely addicted then you will feel little unease at all). The major symptom of this withdrawal will be the actual CRAVING for the substance (or further activity, like gaming machines). Whatever it is, you've either got to eat it, or do it.

Whilst the craving is with you, it will seem as if it is locked in for life. And nothing, absolutely NOTHING, will shift it. Even if you could shift it (you think), it will soon return stronger than ever, and the only way out of this dreadful situation will be to take it again. This is the reason for the failure that is reflected everywhere you look in our modern society: all the fat people licking their ice creams amd smoking their fags. They cannot handle the craving that comes with deprivation of their substance.

But I am going to show you how YOU can handle these withdrawals.

How to Stop Smoking

As doubtless many of my overweight readers will be smokers, this will be of special importance to you. It may be that the chemicals in cigarettes will be other substances to which you are allergic, but as smoking can interfere with pulse readings, and as taking the pulse regularly is part of food allergy testing, commonsense dictates that you must stop the habit. Even if you have failed many times before, in this chapter and the next I can give you invaluable help so that this time you most certainly will do it!

I present you now with the thinking that you must adopt whilst coming off cigarettes.

You should have your last cigarette at night, then go to sleep. When you waken in the morning you will almost certainly want that first cigarette. That is your first craving of the day, which you will feel will NEVER go away unless you satisfy it. With foods, this craving won't necessarily be first thing in the morning and it may not be as strong, but to a degree all this information still applies to the food allergic.

You will certainly not believe it at the time, but that first craving of the day WILL go away, but you must RIDE IT OUT, knowing that once you do ride it out, then it WILL definitely disappear.

That is a promise. However, it will also come back! Then you will once more think that it will never go away. But wrong. Do the same thing: RIDE IT OUT, knowing if you do so, it will definitely go away again. And it will! And so it will go on. Craving first, when you will grit your teeth and RIDE IT OUT, knowing with absolute *certainty* that it will go away. And furthermore you can now be happy with this extra knowledge; the cravings will become slowly weaker and weaker, and the duration in between (where I can assure you, you're NOT craving) will get longer and longer. Until the cravings, which are now not only getting weaker and weaker, but getting shorter and shorter in duration, disappear altogether, with the odd short one rising now and again for a month or two.

Another phenomenon: sometimes these cravings just come out of the blue. But at other times they can be triggered by seeing someone on television lighting up a cigarette or having a huge plate of pasta, or whatever your substance. But here again, the same principle MUST be applied: RIDE IT OUT and it WILL go away! You have now proved to yourself that 'Riding it out' *works*, so that should give you the confidence to keep doing it whenever necessary. Each one will get easier. The hardest 'Riding it out' will always be at the beginning. So, if you can go one *day*, you can go one year, because it gets easier – and that's a fact! And you will NOT be an exception; this applies to everyone!

But beware! Do NOT think, when one of the above scenarios comes into play, for example seeing someone on television lighting up a cigarette, that you can have 'just one' and that will be all and that you won't take any more again. Beware that very common mistake!

Just having the one cigarette, or the one bar of chocolate, still feeds the addiction. It keeps the addiction mechanism simmering. It is a bad move. You MUST, once you are off them, stay off them, unless you want to go over all that again! It's taken you such an effort to do it, and you've succeeded. You've managed to keep away from your favourite or allergic foods that you thought you couldn't live without. You've lost perhaps three or four stones. You've stopped smoking. You are in total control. Don't, for Heaven's sake jeopardise that by doing what you well know is wrong. If you must, have a 'blow out' prior to stopping for good. Know that for a fact, the meal (or cigarettes) you are going to have today – the day before you start your new life – will be your last until your allergies have been sorted out. Do not feel deprived during the blow-out; stuff your face if you feel so inclined, so that tommorrow, when your life starts anew, you will not feel you have been deprived.

How to Test For Tobacco Allergy

You may test yourself for tobacco allergy by stopping smoking for five days and on the fifth day getting someone else to blow cigarette smoke into a cupful of water, until the water turns brown. Put one drop of the liquid under your tongue and slightly tilt your head back. Hold it there for a full minute and a half. If you are allergic to tobacco smoke you should get such a strong reaction that, hopefully, it will put you off the weed for the rest of your days!

The next chapter will be of profound interest to anyone who has ever experienced the cravings that co-exist with withdrawal symptoms. The relatively little-known, but supremely powerful, allies in the battle against addiction are Nature's own willpower-assisters: raw vegetable juices!

SIX

The Miracle Willpower Substitute

Let me now introduce you to the substance that I promise you will actually *endow* you with the willpower that you may need if you prove to be allergic to your favourite food(s):

Raw Vegetable Juices!

By drinking freely of these wonderful enzyme-rich juices, your withdrawal symptoms will be minimal or non-existent, and so too will the cravings that you would normally experience when moving away from the foods you long for. The raw juices actually have an ability to reinforce whatever willpower you have!

It has been found, time and again, particularly on the Gerson Therapy (a dietary therapy for cancer) that many patients have been able to give up smoking with considerable ease, and at least one heroin addict experienced merely a first night's disturbed sleep, thereafter abandoning the drug for good, by taking these wonderful juices.

There is a quality about raw, fresh, organic vegetable juice that has inherent within it some mechanism that quickly corrects, or fights, the craving for substances unnatural to the human system (it is indeed rare to crave foods that are natural – like fruits and vegetables, so I include processed, or refined and even cooked foods, in the 'unnatural' category).

For those of you who may have difficulty in absorbing and assimilating any foodstuffs, there is the added bonus in that the raw juices, with their valuable nutrients, go directly into the bloodstream and are absorbed within 10 to 15 minutes.

In cooked foods, the nutrients are often destroyed, either partially or entirely, by the heat. Certainly the valuable enzymes which are in the foods will be destroyed at temperatures over 118 degrees F. Enzymes are not intended to exist above blood-heat.

If we were Stone Age men, hunting for, say, a sabre-toothed tiger, and were lucky enough to capture one without being eaten ourselves, then the meat we consumed of that tiger would be no warmer than blood heat, and the enzymes would be alive and thus the food would be healthy and natural. Above that blood heat the enzymes begin to be destroyed. It appears everything has to abide by Nature's rules, lest we indeed suffer!

The health benefits that can be derived from drinking raw vegetable juices are almost unbelievable. Dr. Kirschner relates a fascinating story of a baby girl who was born in 1951.[34] At birth she appeared normal but after two months it turned out she had leukaemia. She was taken into hospital and there within the space of five and a half days she was given twenty-five blood transfusions. But all these superhuman efforts to save the child were fruitless, and the little girl died at the age of three months.

The second child, a boy, was born in 1953. On examination, this baby was shown to have been *born with leukaemia*. The baby's doctor had heard about a Mrs Catherine Ferraro, who had recovered from splenic leukaemia by taking large quantities of fresh, raw carrot juice daily. He immediately contacted Mrs Ferraro by telephone, and arranged for her to bring two quarts of carrot juice to the hospital each day. The Ferraros were delighted to comply, and when the baby went home the carrot juice therapy was continued.

It is interesting to note that during the first three months of this baby's life, NO OTHER FOOD was

allowed. After three months however, fruits and vegetables were added to the diet. After one year, the child's
blood count was normal: the leukaemia was gone! Today
(wrote Kirschner in 1956), at the age of five, with the
exception of some occasional asthma, the little fellow is
in apparently perfect health.

The third child, a girl, was born in 1954. Her blood count
was normal. There was no leukaemia. This favourable condition was probably due to the fact that the mother drank
large quantities of carrot juice throughout her pregnancy.
And she fed her third child on nothing but carrot juice
for the first three months of her life, after witnessing her
son's recovery on the same diet.

These juices that have this marvellous effect should
preferably be fresh and not from cans or bottles. They
should be extracted by a machine that grinds the carrots
to extract the juice and not a centrifugal machine. The
canned or bottled juices are an acceptable second choice,
but because of the lack of freshness, they are not our first
choice.

These raw juices are almost entirely used in the nourishment and regeneration of the cells and tissues and
glands and organs within the body. There is another
function, which we cannot explain but which they do
indeed perform; they somehow diminish greatly the
addictive withdrawal state which, as explained before,
is constant in patients who try to change their diet.

The drinking of these vegetable juices conveys instant
nourishment to the nutrition-starved cells within the
refined-food-fed body of the average Briton or American.

And for the allergic fatty, you will find you have the
willpower to remove yourself easily from the foods to
which you are allergic when you might otherwise (if you
didn't have the juices) experience overwhelming urges to
partake of your favourite foods. But with this willpower
aid the entire process will be very much easier than you
had ever hoped.

If you should be unlucky enough to experience any
minor unease or discomfort during the early days, then
drink freely of carrot juice throughout the day and you

will find these feelings will be short-lived. You will soon prove to yourself that for once in your dieting history, YOU and not the food are in control!

And no one will be happier to hear of your success than I. I invite all readers who have success to write to me care of the publishers. It would be a never-ending source of delight to receive such letters!

The quality of the raw vegetable juices is superior in a machine that grinds the juice out of them, such as a Norwalk or a Champion Juicer. Both are expensive, but they are quality machines. They will become heirlooms which you can hand down to your children! Centrifugal machines, in which air has insufficient access to the grinding process, are less desirable.

To quote from Dr. Gerson's book *A Cancer Therapy – Results of Fifty Cases*: 'When the grinding wheel rotates against a resistance with insufficient access of air, positive electricity is produced and induces negative electricity on the surrounding wall. The exchange of the positive and negative electricity kills the oxidizing enzymes and renders the juice deficient.'

Do not, however, despair if you only have a centrifugal machine as there is still sufficient willpower-assisting qualities in such juices to suit the purpose of this book in helping you during the transition period from your old foods to the new. Bottled or canned juice can also be a reasonable second choice and suitable for your purpose, but it would always be better to have the juice fresh. In the early days of your transition, when you may be drinking just the one type of juice – to which you have proven not to be allergic – you can drink as much as 3 or 4 pints a day if necessary! No matter what, should a craving arise, freely sip at the vegetable juices and it will soon go!

The raw juices should be from any of the following vegetables, either singly or mixed, but when taking them you should still monitor your pulse before and after to ensure these are not drinks to which you are allergic.

Preferred Vegetable Juices:
Carrot Beetroot Cabbage Spinach

Carrot Juice

One of the most delicious juices of all the vegetable juices. It helps normalise the entire system. It serves as an aid to digestion. Intestinal and liver diseases are sometimes due to a lack of certain of the elements contained in properly prepared raw carrot juice. When this is the case, then a noticeable cleaning up of the liver may take place, and the material which was clogging it up may be found to dissolve. Frequently this is released so copiously that the intestinal and urinary channels are inadequate to care for this overflow, and in a perfectly natural manner it is passed into the lymph for elimination from the body by means of the pores of the skin. This material has a distinctly orange or yellow pigment and while it is being so eliminated from the body will sometimes discolour the skin. Whenever such a discolouration takes place after drinking carrot or other juices over a period of time, it is an indication that the liver is getting a well-needed cleansing.

It is NOT the carrot juice itself, nor the carotene that comes through the skin, as this discolouration will take place even if the juice is filtered to the point of clearing it of all colour pigment. It is just as practical an impossibility for the carrot pigment itself to come through the skin as it would be for the red pigment of the beetroot juice to turn the body red or the chlorophyll of the green vegetables to paint the skin green from within! Anyway, this yellow discolouration of the skin is a good thing and it is only temporary.

Beetroot Juice

One of the most valuable juices for helping to build up the red corpuscles of the blood and tone up the blood generally. Taken alone, in greater quantities than a wine glass at a time, beetroot juice may cause a cleansing reaction which may make one a little dizzy or nauseated. Therefore reduce the beetroot or mix with a larger quantity of carrot juice until you can tolerate the beneficial cleansing effect.

Cabbage Juice

Some people find it difficult to drink this raw, but it is excellent mixed with carrot juice. Duodenal ulcers have responded almost miraculously to the drinking of cabbage juice. Such is the quality of raw cabbage juice, properly prepared, that the drinking of a mere half pint provides more vital organic food value that is assimilated by the body than one hundred and twenty pounds in weight of cooked or canned cabbage! Cabbage juice has been shown in double-blind trials, when the effects were tested against a placebo, to reduce the pain of, and speed up the healing process in, stomach uclers.[35]

Spinach Juice

Spinach is the most vital food for the entire digestive tract, both the alimentary section of the body (the stomach, duodenum, and small intestines) and for the large intestine or colon, and it has been so recognised from time immemorial.

You can mix these juices as and how you please, according to taste, but most people prefer carrot juice to be the major constituent, with smaller quantities of the others. You may find that carrot juice entirely on its own is your favourite – it's up to you. If you only have carrots in the house, fine, but it is generally best to add the extra juices in from time to time.

As a basis for good health, it is best to take upwards of one pint of raw vegetable juice daily. As a normal tumbler is approximately half a pint, it is not difficult to consume one pint per day. For controlling cravings, if you have to go to work, although not preferred over freshly made juice, you should take enough juice to last you, in a flask: these will see you through any difficult times whilst you are changing your diet.

SEVEN

Case Histories

The following patients did not seek help solely for their weight problems; they had other health disorders as well as their overweight.

Case No. 1

Patient:	Mr. M.A.
Age:	56
Occupation:	Therapist
Symptoms:	Obesity, lethargy, loss of self confidence.
Treatment:	Food allergy detection and avoidance.
Weight loss on treatment:	Still losing.

Comments: Patient couldn't resist many foods such as toast, scones and teacakes. All were based on wheat. For ten days patient had all he wanted to eat except foods containing wheat. He enjoyed beef with gravy, but no Yorkshire pudding, fish, and chips without any batter on the fish, ham, bacon, eggs, cheese, vegetables, fruit, butter and grains other than wheat. Breakfast was a large bowl of porridge. He was never hungry but did experience headaches on the first two days and a groggy, irritable, restless feeling persisted until about day 5. Then the clouds lifted. By the time the ten days were up, M.A. returned feeling more energetic, wearing a bright shirt and looking very well indeed. He had lost the puffiness in his face. He had lost 7 lbs in the ten days and is still losing. He no longer has food cravings. Patient delighted!

Case No. 2:

Patient:	Mrs C.E.
Age:	55
Occupation:	Housewife
Symptoms	M.E., Overweight.
Treatment:	Food allergy detection and avoidance.
Weight loss on treatment:	3 stones.

Comments: Had a 'viral' complaint since 1977 but it was not recognised as M.E. until 1990. Tested for food allergies and found to be allergic to cheese, eggs, wheat and cucumber amongst others. By avoidance lost all M.E. symptoms and delighted at losing 3 stones in under 5 months.

Case No. 3

Patient:	Mr. M.F.
Age:	15
Occupation:	Student
Symptoms:	Severe Asthma. Overweight. Unable to attend school.
Treatment:	Food allergy detection and avoidance.
Weight loss on treatment:	1 stone.

Comments: Proved allergic to tobacco smoke, house dust mite, wheat, cat hair, chicken, sunflower oil, tap water. Homeopathic desensitisation marginally improved symptoms. Return to school worsened asthma; transpired allergic to chalk! After removal of allergens all symptoms cleared up. Weight normalised and martial arts became a passion.

Case No. 4

Patient:	Dr. W.
Age:	75
Occupation:	Retired medical doctor.
Symptoms:	Severe asthma, sinusitis, rhinorrhea (nasal discharge). Overweight.
Treatment:	Food/chemical allergy detection and avoidance.
Weight loss on treatment:	2 stones +

Comments: All symptoms cleared by avoiding foods and chemicals to which he was sensitive and his weight normalised for first time in many years. Patient is a retired medical doctor who, in his later years, turned to food allergy detection (clinical ecology) and is now a fully-fledged clinical ecologist. Says if he could have his time over again his first chosen method of treatment would undoubtedly be diet.

Case No. 5

Patient:	Miss S.E.
Age:	46
Occupation:	Secretary
Symptoms:	Some overweight, irritability, breathlessness, constipation, bouts of anger.
Treatment:	Food allergy detection and avoidance.
Weight loss on treatment:	7lbs

Comments: Patient had symptoms for over two years and although visited doctor, had no joy. Irritable bowel syndrome diagnosed. Found to be allergic to eggs and coffee. Reported feeling 'marvellous' at end of first week. Lost her 7lbs overweight at which she was thrilled, along with all her other symptoms.

Case No. 6

Patient:	Miss L.B.
Age:	75
Occupation:	Retired.
Symptoms:	Overweight, constant hay fever symptoms, watery eyes and runny nose.
Treatment:	Food allergy detection and avoidance.
Weight loss on treatment:	8lbs

Comments: Suffered symptoms for 30–40 years. After avoidance of dairy products and alcohol, to which she was allergic, all her symptoms vanished in two weeks, with her stubborn overweight finally disappearing. So thoroughly delighted she recommended almost 50 other patients for the treatment!

Case No. 7

Patient:	Mr. D.
Age:	31
Occupation:	Catering Manager
Symptoms:	Overweight, itchy scalp (very raw) with severe dandruff.
Treatment:	Food allergy detection and avoidance.
Weight loss on treatment:	1 stone

Comments: Patient suffered from stubborn overweight for years and had a very itchy and inflamed scalp with heavy dandruff. Proved to be allergic to salt, fat and chocolate. After avoiding these substances, his scalp greatly improved after few weeks, all dandruff cleared and he lost his one stone overweight.

Case No. 8

Patient:	Mr. R.H.
Age:	46
Occupation:	Businessman
Symptoms:	Obesity, depression, irritability,

insomnia, lethargy

Treatment: Food allergy detection and avoidance.

Weight loss
on treatment: 4 stones

Comments: Patient suffered from obesity for many years along with other annoying symptoms for which he had seen a psychiatrist. The psychiatrist, although a good listener, was useless at actually helping his symptoms. Tested for food allergies and found to have multiple sensitivities to alcohol, tobacco and other refined foods. On avoiding the substances all his mental symptoms cleared up and his weight just seemed to 'pour' off. He was absolutely delighted, as he had previously thought he would have to feel miserable for the rest of his days!

Case No. 9

Patient: Miss S.
Age: Fortysomething.
Occupation: Secretary
Symptoms: Obesity, lack of coordination, fatigue
Treatment: Food allergy detection and avoidance.

Weight loss
on treatment: 2 stones

Comments: Patient suffered from obscure feelings of lack of coordination and constant fatigue. Given drugs by her doctor which did no good at all. By reading food allergy book she recognised she was likely food allergic. By avoiding whole grains and meat to which she proved allergic, all her symptoms cleared up and she lost two stone.

Case No. 10

Patient: Mrs R.H.
Age: 44
Occupation: Housewife
Symptoms: Overweight, headache with blurred vision, constant fatigue.

Treatment: Food allergy detection and avoidance.
Weight loss
on treatment: 2½ stones

Comments: Patient had suffered headache and blurred vision for 8 years, since the birth of her second baby. The overweight stemmed from the same time. Doctor had advised her she had migraine and gave her drugs, which did no good at all. Found to be allergic to coffee, alcohol, cheese, eggs, and most tinned soups. After removal of these items from her diet, she reported being headache and blurred-vision free for the first time in years after only a week. Her fatigue lifted soon after and she lost all her overweight.

EIGHT

Avoiding Further Reactions: The Rotation Diet

If you follow the instructions in this book, you should be able to identify the foods/drinks/chemicals to which you are allergic, and by avoiding them, remain slim – and symptom-free if you have symptoms. However, there are a number of less lucky individuals, who, even when clear of their allergenic foods, can, by repeated eating of a food to which they are NOT allergic, create an allergy to that food. They can, by repeated exposure, become sensitised to it.

Most food allergies are cyclic; you are not born with them but develop them with repeated exposure to the foods. In these cyclic allergies, if you do not consume the food for a lengthy period, you may well be able to eat it again without harm. But you should not repeatedly then eat it or you may run the risk of stirring up the allergy again.

And some people can develop new sensitivities merely by repeatedly eating the same food – even if they think they are eating non-allergenic foods.

To avoid the possibility of new allergies surfacing, a Rotation Diet can be followed with great success. This involves the spacing out of foods so that you do not become sensitive to them. The most effective approach is not to consume the food more than once in every four days. You may eat as much as you wish of that food, as long as it is – ideally – at the ONE SITTING. I will give you an example of a Rotation Diet below. The modern

Rotation Diet is based on an early form of rotation diet developed by Dr. Herbert Rinkel of Kansas City, who back in the 1930s developed the Rotary Diversified Diet.

It should be pointed out, too, that another phenomenon which can plague the allergy sufferer is that even by only eating a food once in every four days, there is still a possibility of developing a new allergy to that food if he consumes other foods from the same food FAMILY on a regular basis. I give below the Food Families and an example of a Rotation Diet:

Example of Four Day Rotation Diet
Day 1: Apple Juice. Eggs. Chicken. Lettuce. Carrot. Carrot Juice. Celery. Apples. Pears. Pomegranate.
Day 2: Orange Juice. Milk. Beef. Cauliflower. Cabbage. Brussel Sprouts. Tuna. Oranges. Peas. Beans. Hazelnuts.
Day 3: Grape Juice. Haddock. Potato. Tomatoes. Grapes. Cucumber. Sultanas. Melon. Beetroot. Brazil Nuts.
Day 4: Pineapple Juice. Bananas. Buckwheat. Salmon. Trout. Brown Rice. Mushrooms. Onions. Leeks.

Of course you would find out whether or not you were allergic to any of the above before including them in your diet. You may make up your own diet based on the understanding that you do not repeat the same food family until four days have lapsed. Here is a list of food families. Remember, if you are to consume more than one member of the same food family, do so on the same day; preferably even in the same hour. (Those foods which are marked 'single' have no other foods in the same family.)

Plant Food Families Alphabetically by Food Name

Food	Family Name	Food	Family Name
alfalfa	legume	cantaloupe	gourd
almond	plum	caraway	parsley
allspice	myrtle	carob	legume
anise	parsley	carrot	parsley
apple	apple	cashew	cashew
apricot	plum	cauliflower	mustard
arrowroot	single	cayenne	potato
artichoke,		celery	parsley

common		celery cabbage	mustard
globe		chard, Swiss	beet
Jerusalem	single	cherry	plum
asparagus	lily	chestnut	single
avocado	laurel	chicory	composite
banana	banana	chilli	potato
barley	cereal	chives	lily
basil	mint	chocolate	stercula
bay leaf	laurel	cinnamon	laurel
beans	legume	citron	citrus
beet	beet	clove	myrtle
blackberry	rose	cocoa	stercula
blueberry	heather	coconut	palm
boysenberry	rose	coffee	single
brazil nut	single	cola	stercula
broccoli	mustard	collard	mustard
Brussels		coriander	parsley
sprouts	mustard	corn	cereal
buckwheat	buckwheat	cottonseed	mallow
butternut	walnut	cranberry	heather
cabbage	mustard	cucumber	gourd
currant	gooseberry	molasses	cereal
dandelion	composite	mulberry	mulberry
date	palm	mushroom	fungus
dewberry	rose	muskmelon	gourd
dill	parsley	mustard	mustard
eggplant	potato	nectarine	plum
elderberry	single	nutmeg	nutmeg
endive	composite	oat	cereal
escarole	composite	okra	mallow
fennel	parsley	olive	single
fig	mulberry	onion	lily
filbert	single	orange	citrus
garlic	lily	oregano	mint
ginger	ginger	papaya	single
ginseng	single	paprika	potato
gooseberry	gooseberry	parsley	parsley
grape	single	parsnip	parsley
grapefruit	citrus	pea	legume
green pepper	potato	peach	plum
guava	myrtle	peanut	legume
hazelnut	single	pear	apple
hickory	walnut	pecan	walnut
hop	mulberry	pepper black	single
horehound	mint	white	
horseradish	mustard	pepper green	potato
huckleberry	heather	red	
Jerusalem		peppermint	mint
artichoke	composite	pineapple	single

kale	mustard	pine nut	single
kohlrabi	mustard	pistachio	cashew
kumquat	citrus	plantain	banana
leek	lily	plum	plum
lemon	citrus	pomegranate	single
lentil	legume	potato	potato
lettuce	composite	prune	plum
licorice	legume	pumpkin	gourd
lime	citrus	quince	apple
loganberry	rose	radish	mustard
macadamia nut	single	raisin	single
mace	nutmeg	raspberry	rose
malt	cereal	red pepper	potato
mango	cashew	rhubarb	buckwheat
maple	single	rice	cereal
marjoram	mint	rutabaga	mustard
melons	gourd	rye	cereal
millet	cereal	sage	mint
mint	mint	sago	palm
safflower	composite	thyme	mint
salsify	composite	tobacco	potato
savory	mint	tomato	potato
sesame	single	tumeric	ginger
soybean	legume	turnip	mustard
spearmint	mint	vanilla	single
spinach	beet	walnut	walnut
squash	gourd	water chestnut	single
strawberry	rose	watercress	mustard
sugar cane	cereal	watermelon	gourd
sunchoke	sunflower	wheat	cereal
sweet potato	single	wild rice	cereal
tangerine	citrus	wintergreen	heather
tapioca	single	yam	single
tea	single	yeast	fungus

(Note: The yam is a tropical plant that is in a different family from the sweet potato.)

Animal Food Families

Bovines:	Cattle (beef), milk and dairy products, goat, mutton, lamb.
Poultry:	Chicken, eggs, pheasant, quail.
Swine:	Bacon, ham, lard, pork, pork scratchings.
Duck:	Duck, goose.
Flatfish:	Dab, flounder, halibut, plaice, sole, turbot.
Salmon:	Salmon, trout.

Mackerel: Bonito, mackerel, skipjack, tuna.
Codfish: Cod, coley, haddock, hake, ling.
Herring: Herring, pilchard, rollmop, sardine.
Molluscs: Abalone, clam, mussel, oyster, scallop, snail, squid.
Crustaceans: Crab, crayfish, lobster, prawn, shrimp.

It may be that you will never need to use these Food Family lists. You may be one of the fortunates who can quickly get rid of their surplus weight or symptoms by mere avoidance of certain foods. But should you get into difficulty, with a new allergy surfacing, simply start monitoring your pulse whilst writing down any symptoms you may experience. It will soon become obvious if there is another allergen in your diet. If you get in a muddle, simply go back to testing one food at a time until you get a clear picture of which is the offending food and cut it out entirely. And rotate your other foods for a while until you are clear of all symptoms and you have your confidence in the technique restored.

NINE

Obesity as a Health Problem

Interest in obesity as a health problem began at the start of the century with studies conducted by American insurance companies. These culminated in the 1959 Build and Blood Pressure Study, in which the experience of minimum mortality led to the publication of the famous tables of 'desirable weights'. Evidence has now accumulated in the scientific literature of adverse medical and psychological consequences of being overweight and its effect on longevity.[36]

Obesity can be defined as adiposity (excessive accumulation of fat within the body) in excess of that consistent with health, or more regularly recognised as 20 per cent over your ideal weight for your height.

At age 25 the normal amount of fat at what is termed 'desirable' weight is about 14 percent of body weight for males and 25 percent for females. These figures tend to rise in later years, even when the weight remains constant.

In recent years the measurement of skinfold thickness has been introduced as a relatively simple method for estimating the body fat. A triceps skinfold thickness equal to, or greater than, 23mm in man and 30 mm in women between the ages of 30 and 50 is an indicator of obesity.

Life assurance company tables that give the ideal weight for a given height based on mortality data for various height-weight groups are of some value. These tables for 25 year olds can be used as ideal standards throughout life, as the ideal weight for adults of all ages corresponds to the actual weight at 25.

However, in recent years Assurance companies have increased their estimates of 'average' weights by approximately ten per cent, so it seems even they can get it wrong!

It has been estimated that between 7 and 25 percent of peoples in affluent societies are obese.

Obese patients are poorer surgical risks than the non-obese. They tend to be clumsy and more accident prone. Whilst obesity is not responsible for initiating certain disease processes it does tend to unmask or enhance these and conversely, if treated, contributes to amelioration of the underlying conditions. Among these may be included diabetes, possibly hypertension (high blood pressure) and bone, joint and muscle diseases. Extreme obesity increases the work of breathing, decreases respiratory reserve and maximum capacity, and causes changes in the circulation contributing to dyspnoea (difficulty in, or laboured breathing).[37]

Although the observation that extreme obesity affects respiratory function is not new, a disorder of breathing during sleep has relatively recently been suggested as a complication of excessive fatness.[38]

A study of 20 overweight and 20 normal volunteers during sleep gave a clear insight into this transitory, but frightening, stopping of breathing during sleep. Apnoea was defined as a pause in airflow for more than ten seconds. The obese patients with sleep apnoea showed the greatest disturbance of sleep and generally slept the shortest time. Although the obese patients showed a higher incidence of sleep apnoea, not all obese volunteers experienced them, and besides, a few of the normal weight volunteers suffered mild cessation of breathing during the study.

As the research showed, this frightening stopping of breathing was indeed more evident in the fat person, yet it was not exclusively a fat individual's complaint.

The possibility of some ingredient in the patients' evening meals being contributory to the symptoms was never considered. And as fat people are certainly food allergic, then the possibility should have been an important consideration, as food allergy reactions can show up as almost any disorder.

Incidence of abnormal liver function readings, generally thought to be the result of alcoholism, has been shown to be prevalent in obese non-drinkers.[39] This indicates that a diet of refined, processed – and almost certainly allergenic – foods, when consumed by the obese person, can in itself cause liver function abnormalities and should not be immediately thought by doctors to be the result of alcoholic over-indulgence. In a group of obese individuals, liver biopsies showed it to be damaged in every single case, and not one had abnormal liver function.[40,41,42]

A study of breast-fed infants showed that these children are leaner than formula-fed children. Another way of reading the result of that trial would be that breast-fed children will not be ingesting foods to which they are likely to be allergic, thus the normal weight, whilst the non-breast fed child may indeed be consuming foods to which he is reacting.

Earlier studies of breast-feeding were inconclusive as the trials only lasted about 4–6 months, but a new one year study which concluded that breast-fed children were indeed leaner was recently carried out. The trial's definition of breast-fed included only those who received breast milk as the sole source of milk throughout the first year of life. Thus, they concluded, the duration of breast feeding may be a key variable influencing infant fatness.[43]

There have been studies which have shown that obesity can be the result of a stressful life event.[44] Other research has also provided evidence of obesity being associated with traumatic events. But you should remember that allergies, or the allergic capability, can lie dormant for years and only surface after a traumatic event whether a bereavement, or financial distress, or indeed a bodily injury, such as the result of a car crash. Therefore, both the allergic syndrome and the pattern of obesity can appear as one after such an event, yet the obesity awareness of the patient would be the only noticeable change. Unless he knew of the food allergy concept, he would not be aware of the link between his obesity and possible allergenic substances in his diet.

Obesity carries an increased risk of several serious diseases such as hypertension, coronary heart disease, cerebral stroke, and diabetes mellitus, and is associated with increased mortality.[45-50]

The heart, liver, joints, kidneys and circulation can all be adversely affected by excess weight. Even the colon (the large bowel) can, when large amounts of unnatural, processed foods and chemicals are pushed into it, suffer, and can often become twisted, with possible serious complications.

Another research group investigating the long-term effects of reducing was unable to find persons who had reduced and maintained normal weight so they were forced to use rats. The animals on a diet of natural foods ate all they wanted and kept in excellent health without gaining weight,[51] which suggests to me that the natural-food fed rats were not creating deficiencies within themselves by their unrefined diets, which would lead to the allergic syndrome.

The view, commonly held, that all obese people overeat has not been substantiated by several surveys. It was found that obese school children actually ate less than their normal weight controls but spent very much less of their time in activities involving exercise.[52]

In another study, 31 obese and 31 normal weight children matched for age and sex were measured for physical fitness using a two-stage exercise test on a bicycle ergometer.[63]

The obese children were physically less fit than the normal weight subjects as judged from the pedalling time in the exercise test. The observation that obese children are less fit favours the concept that obese children are underactive as compared with normal weight children.[54] The conclusion was that the reduction in fitness seemed to be related to the degree of obesity.

Other surveys however have indicated further conclusions, with some of which I would most certainly not agree.

It has been suggested that because the obese child is less likely to take part in sports, therefore that lack of involvement was contributory to the obesity of the child.

But the true picture is somewhat less confusing to the Clinical Ecologist. If the child eats foods to which he is unwittingly allergic, then his glands will undoubtedly malfunction, interfering with his metabolism, which will result in overweight.

Such overweight will decrease oxygen consumption in the child whilst undertaking physical activity, which will further inhibit his performance and will result in his reluctance to take part altogether, or only at a very limited level. This does not take into account the very high possibility that, included within the allergic reaction to foods, will be an element of fatigue contraindicating physical activity. Such inactivity will then compound the obesity factor and so the never-ending cycle carries on.

The only way to break it would be to test the child and ascertain his food allergens and remove them. The resultant weight loss and removal of possible fatigue will restore his desire to take part in physical activity and Eureka – the cycle will have ceased.

So whilst two schoolchildren may eat identical diets and one piles the weight on whilst his pal stays skinny, it has little to do with the *amount* of food eaten, but the way the children's bodies handle the foods. The fat child has a slow metabolism because of the allergic food items slowing down his thyroid function whilst the thin child eats foods which speed up his metabolism.

TEN

Other Methods of Weight Loss

Exercise

Practically useless! You need to burn up an amazing 3,500 calories simply to lose one pound in weight! You would have to saw wood non-stop for twelve hours to burn off that solitary pound, or, if you preferred, swim non-stop for 12 hours, or walk – again non-stop – for 12 solid hours!

Exercise is vital for promoting health but in itself pretty hopeless as a weight loss regimen. If you are fat just now and have no energy, do not worry as, when you lose your weight by removing the allergenic foods, your energy will also return.

I often see obese people pounding the streets as a means of trying to get themselves 'into shape' and I often wonder if they KNOW that, although charging round the streets may seem to them a pretty positive approach to healthier living, it will do almost nothing for the massive weight they are carrying! They have to attend to the other part of the problem; what they stuff into themselves.

Stomach stapling

Life-threatening obesity justifies treatment by surgery, according to the authors of one study,[55] provided that the risk of operating does not exceed the risk of the condition itself.

Morbid obesity is defined as greater than 100 percent excess weight. The obesity itself is only rarely the immediate or sole cause of illness or death. Localised fat can cause obstruction and/or organ compression resulting in clinical disorders. Most of the obesity-associated risk factors, as well as the indicated disease conditions discussed earlier in this book, interact to (a) diminish quality of life; (b) impair health, and (c) shorten survival.

Gastroplasty is a method whereby the stomach capacity is reduced considerably by means of surgical stapling.

Over 90 percent of the weight loss occurs in the first year, with slight tendency to weight gain at 18, 24 and 30 months.

There can be postoperative complications in about 1 in 5 cases, with symptoms varying from vomiting to staple-line disruption. One case of death was recorded in a study of 300 patients.

Jaw Wiring

Weight loss pattern was analysed in 26 grossly overweight patients after jaw fixation. During an average fixation time of 7 months, the average weight loss in females was almost 20kg (just over three stones) and in males 30kg (4½ stones). Two years after fixation, the average weight loss in women was 13.8kg (just over two stones). A psychiatric followup revealed that most patients reported moderate psychiatric symptoms during treatment. Patients reporting that they ate for consolation tended to regain weight after fixation, whereas patients not reporting this eating pattern continued to lose weight.[56]

Very-Low-Calorie-Diets (VLCDs)

The treatment of obesity by normal low calorie diets can be difficult and often discouraging because the failure rate is very high. Even with success, the average long-term weight loss is modest.

It is because of the rather dismal results with conventional low caloric diets that the very-low-calorie diets (VLCDs) have gained enormous favour in the past fifteen or so years. Because the VLCDs are severely limited in calories (300–600 calories per day) a large energy deficit occurs, with weight losses in the range of 18–22kg in 12–15 weeks and 30–35kg in 25 weeks. These diets are easy to use and require little effort from either the patient or the health professional. And since the formulae contain high quality protein and appropriate vitamins and minerals they are considered to be relatively safe.

Although VLCDs were introduced as early as 1929 in America, they became truly popular in the 1970s. Since then there has been recurrent controversy over their safety and composition.

There are financial-ethical questions to the VLCD business. There is always a possible conflict of interest when selling a product as a treatment modality. There may be a strong temptation to continue to prescribe the products – to continue to reap the profits from the product. It was for this reason that, years ago, the United States prohibited physicians from having their own pharmacies and making profits on the medication they prescribed. The unconscionable length of time that many patients are being kept on VLCDs even nowadays may in great part be related to this. Profits drive many programmes, not necessarily what is best for the patients.[57]

Fasting as a Means of Weight Loss and Restoring Health

I want to discuss fasting here as it is a common method employed by many food allergic people who, by avoiding for a period of four or five days all foods, will experience a clear-cut reaction upon eating foods that affect them. It is a diagnostic tool with a high level of accuracy. Although all foodstuffs are avoided, bottled drinking water must be taken, as, although man can live many weeks without food, he can go without water for only a few days.

The faster, during his four or five days' avoidance, becomes sensitised to all foods and it is this super-sensitivity that makes the technique so reliable for identifying culprit foods or drinks.

Fasting is also the quickest and surest way to lose weight. And the weight loss can be nothing short of remarkable.

There have been many studies in fasting,[58–61] and total fasting for the treatment of severely obese patients has been frequently used in the past.

The impressive loss of bodyweight (initially often huge water losses) can streamline a person's body and face in anything from a few days to a few weeks, dependent of course upon the amount you have to lose – and the amount of allergic oedema that exists within your body. This allergic oedema is noticeable on puffy, pasty-like faces that are commonplace nowadays and these features can 'tighten' quite dramatically after only a few days. This comes as a result not only of the fasting, but of the removal of the allergenic foods which can cause such puffiness.

Although some people have been known to fast for anything up to 90 days, anything longer than 7 days should be under the care of a practitioner experienced in fasting, and it is not recommended as a do-it-yourself treatment, as complications can arise that need expert assessment. Professor Ditschuneit of the University Clinic of Ulm has written:[62] 'The human body is in a position, because of special regulating mechanisms, to survive complete abstinence from food for many weeks without damaging its health. During a fast the protein loss is reduced to a minimum and strict fasting treatments are effective and carry no risk.'

You can lose up to 20lbs on a 7-day fast, and some people have lost 5lbs on a one-day fast. A loss of 10lbs on a weekend fast is not unusual.

The very thought of fasting would put the fear of death into many people who are unaware of the benefits. But the truth of the matter is, it is quite simple, and even the greediest of people, with only an elementary amount of willpower, can fast for several days, without any discomfort whatsoever. In fact many people want to *continue* fasting because they feel so well. This partly will be because they are removed from the foods to which they are allergic, and the relief to the system can be tremendous. Fasting is easier than going on a low calorie diet because there is no hunger! After about 48 hours, all sensation of hunger disappears. You are not hungry.

This might sound like the very opposite of what would be expected, but it is a well-known phenomenon.

Whilst you are not eating, the body first of all uses up all the carbohydrate stored within the system. Only when the carbohydrates are fully used up (after approximately 48 hours) does the body start to plunder the reserves stored within your body and burn up the fat.

When the body starts that activity – burning up the fat – it burns off ketone bodies; you will be in a state of ketosis, and your breath will unfortunately smell bad. When the breath eventually returns to a sweet smell, that is often accompanied by a return of real, true hunger, and that is the indication for the fast to be broken. But that will take normally several weeks. When you fast, the energies of the body, which are normally involved in digestion and excretion, are solely directed into the excretory part of the work. All energies are then utilised in the sole activity of getting rid of all the wastes the body will have accumulated over the years.

This not inconsiderable work may incur cleansing symptoms – anything from headaches to a fever. But generally these signs are good; they indicate the body still has the vitality actually to do this work!

The difference between starving and fasting is quite distinct. The body has food reserves within it. Whilst fasting these reserves are mobilised for food and, only when all the fat and reserves and waste products are completely used – after anywhere from 3 weeks to as long as (in some cases) 90-odd days, does the body actually start to 'eat itself'.

At this 'cannibalistic' stage the unimportant tissues of the body are used as food, and some remarkable inner intelligence of the body seems to leave the vital organs such as the heart, brain, etc., to the very end in order to preserve life for as long as possible! Of course I am talking about *months* without food and such a scenario as above would only be seen in someone intent on killing himself.

Although fasting is an absolutely excellent method of losing weight for the majority of us, and there is the real added benefit of old toxic accumulations which have been building up in our bodies for years being expelled in the process, it is essential that much preparation be given and careful thought on the actual return to eating!

There was one, admittedly extremely rare, case of a teenage girl a few years ago in England who fasted (water only) for about 4 days and who immediately broke it by gorging with a ridiculous amount of meat and foods of all sorts. According to the newspaper reports her stomach burst open. She died of course, but I emphasise, although it was an extremely rare case, much care has to be applied to the breaking of the fast proper.

The breaking of the fast should ideally be with fruits and/or vegetables and, as a drink, vegetable juice (after the foods). This is nature's food and, depending upon which fasting book you read, the method of breaking the fast will differ quite dramatically. One early Hygienist (naturopath) used to recommend popcorn! But I'm sure that in his time, popcorn was probably a more back-to-nature item than it is today!

Some remarkable and dramatic recoveries from symptoms of many years' standing have resulted from fasting, and it is a wondrous opportunity, if the circumstances are right, for total rejuvenation of the system. But ideally one should be in a fasting institution, and under expert care from someone experienced in long fasts.

For several years Russian psychiatrists have been reporting successful use of prolonged fasts in the treatment of schizophrenia.[63] At the Moscow Psychiatric Institute, Dr. Yuri Nikolayev has fasted many schizophrenics. The patients had been chronically ill and felt hopeless about the future. Many would have lived out the balance of their lives in the bleak wards of mental hospitals. *Seventy* percent of those treated by fasting improved so remarkably that they were able to resume an active life! One such patient at the Institute was a nuclear scientist whose case was diagnosed as senile psychosis. His memory had lapsed to the point where he could not recall his own name. But after an extended fast his memory was completely restored and he regained full possession of his intellectual powers. Most fasts at the Moscow Institute lasted for 25 days.

PART II

What to do about Your Food Allergies

ELEVEN

The Cause of Allergies and What We Can Do About Them

If you have proven to yourself, by using the information in this book, that you have food allergies, what can you do about it?

Certainly, you could dodge the offending foods for the rest of your life if you wish. Or it may be that you have many food allergies and this will prove more difficult than it sounds.

The reason that you are allergic in the first place is due to a faulty nutritional history; whether your own, or your parents' or both. Let the story of Pottenger's Cats explain why this should be:

Pottenger's Cats: An Hereditary Eye-Opener

Francis M. Pottenger M.D., was an American doctor who made significant contributions to the role nutrition plays in maintaining good health, and indeed correcting ill-health.

His classic ten-year study of 900 cats gave a priceless insight into the consequences of poor nutrition upon health, and probably more importantly, on the effect of nutrition on the health of the offspring of the cats.

He fed one group of cats on pasteurised (heated) milk, cooked meat and cod liver oil. These animals developed allergies, were generally in poor health, and had skeletal deformities as well as exhibiting homosexual tendencies.

Further, each successive generation became poorer in health, producing smaller and weaker litters with low birth weight animals.

He fed another group of cats with the same food but this time the meat was raw and the milk UNpasteurised (raw). These animals were healthy, had good skeletal structure and were normal and happy in their behaviour. There was no homosexuality and their offspring too were healthy through successive generations, unlike the cooked-food group which showed all manner of disease symptoms.[64]

Pottenger states: 'In giving cats cooked meat and milk, they develop all kinds of allergies. They sneeze, wheeze and scratch. They are irritable, nervous and do not purr. First deficient generation allergic cats produce second generation kittens with greater incidence of allergies, and by the third generation, the incidence is almost 100 percent.'[65]

This should therefore indicate to the reader the cause of allergies. Effectively, it comes down to poor nutrition. The study also implies nervousness and general irritability is down to nutritional influences. Psychiatrists have spent countless years searching for the elusive key to emotional and mental health; they should look no longer! Those experiments also indicate the extremely controversial possibility that even our sexuality may be dictated – or influenced – by historical nutritional abnormalities.

The Pottenger study clearly shows the link between diet and the health of the parent and ultimately the health of the offspring. And the role nutrition plays in that link. Good nutrition therefore is vital; in cats, snails, tadpoles, baboons, bats, elephants, kangaroos and every other living thing on this planet, including plants, which derive their nutrition from the soil. So it stands to reason, that man should not be an exception. The foods man eats should have as much bearing on his health, and the health of his offspring, as do the foods of other species on their own health.

Most doctors pooh-pooh the suggestion that diet is linked to health and indeed, ill-health. They constantly demand 'proof'. Because they are not taught the connection at Medical School they seem reluctant, or embarrassed, to accept a 'new' theory, especially when it is as stunningly successful as nutritional medicine. Even when presented with proof, many will still endeavour to pass it off as meaningless rather than accept something which poses (they may consider) a threat to their very existence.

There is more proof – more evidence – that changing nutrition can restore health and prevent ill-health, than all the other 'alternative medicine' therapies put together. Doctors often claim the 'placebo' effect has restored patients' health when presented with a recovered patient (through diet). Were Pottenger's cats subject to suggestion; subject to the placebo effect? Were McCarrison's rats who got well on improved nutrition merely getting better because of the placebo effect? Were all the patients, who by intensive, improved nutrition on the Gerson Therapy and who could show before and after X-rays to substantiate their improved health also merely imagining their recovered health? Somehow I doubt it!

For those of you with food allergies, improved nutrition is the only alternative to forever dodging your allergenic foods if mere avoidance of them over a period of time shows no improvement in the allergic condition.

The next chapter will show you just what wonderful health benefits can be achieved by applying intensive nutritional measures, such as that employed by the Gerson Therapy.

TWELVE

The Fantastic Healing Power Within All of Us

It would be a foolish person who did not acknowledge that the body has a wonderful ability to heal itself. All doctors recognise this fact and it is one of the most amazing of all the physiological processes that take place in our bodies. We have come to take the sight of a cut healing for granted; as we do breathing. But the phenomenon itself has been little explored and almost no attention has been paid to the possibility of actually being able to *enhance* this wonderful natural process by the application of super-nutrition. It has little been considered that perhaps poor diet results in a *reduced* healing ability, lending itself to diseases taking 'root'.

By the application of a totally natural diet of fruits, vegetables and nuts, and the entire removal from one's diet of all processed, packaged and tinned foods, all manner of diseases and ill health can be eliminated, including what many of you may not consider 'ill health' at all: overweight. But the fact that your thyroid gland is adversely reacting to the incoming food items at all, indicates a dysfunction, which in turn means – whether you like it or not – that you have less-than-perfect health.

The food-allergic syndrome is one disorder that responds positively to a vastly improved diet. As you have now proven to yourself you are 'allergic', you can remove this allergic state completely with the entire restoration of your health by the application of sound – and sustained – nutritional principles.

This elimination of the allergic syndrome comes about with a regeneration of the entire system by improvement in your nutrition. But needless to say, if you go back to your old nutritional habits too soon, any improvement will be wiped out.

By changing your diet – and sustaining the change for a couple of years – to a totally natural one, abundant in nature's own vitamin and mineral-rich fruits and vegetables, raw juices and nuts or seeds, your state of health can improve dramatically, and symptoms which may have dogged you for years can be eliminated. Nature Cure history abounds with examples of seemingly miraculous cures but which are oftentimes dismissed by doctors as 'spontaneous remission' (in other words, it would have gone away by itself anyway...).

For those of you who have never heard of diet being used to actually *heal* an illness or disorder, let me make one thing quite clear ... It is not a crank notion. It is certainly not new. It has been part of healing for centuries. By application of the correct diet all sorts of disorders can be permanently removed.

However, with the advent of 'miracle' drugs, which influenced (however temporarily) the patients' symptoms, diet was more or less abandoned as the way to heal, in favour of these seemingly miraculous compounds. Drugs acted quickly whilst diet was often slow (but sure).

Nowadays it is becoming increasingly clear that drugs are NOT the answer. Except for some life-saving injections of synthetic hormones such as adrenaline or insulin, the vast majority of drugs merely alleviate – on a temporary basis – the symptom, and almost certainly add a toxic load to the already ill patient's system, without ever actually doing anything about the CAUSE.

They may give the *illusion* of healing, but they never actually *heal*. They may influence the site of the disorder; they may stifle the symptoms and *seemingly* cure the problem, but often the symptom will either return later, or the complaint would have cleared up by the body's own natural healing power anyway.

Doctors are taught next to nothing about nutrition and health at medical school. They are drug orientated.

Let us see an example of how little they consider the average patient's diet as being a factor in their symptoms.

Let us imagine someone living on nothing but jelly babies for an entire year. An unlikely event, I'll admit, but we are only making an example. The patient, after that time, will inevitably (if he is still alive of course) be suffering from all manner of complaints: fatigue, depression, bad skin, to name a few.

Now let our man go to the doctor, complaining of bad skin, fatigue and depression. What will happen? He will doubtless walk out of the surgery clutching prescriptions for all sorts of drugs: drugs for his skin complaint, drugs for his fatigue, and drugs for his depression, when all the time his complaints were dietarily induced. The doctor will not have even considered his diet!

Yet take an exotic animal, say a snake, to a vet, and the first thing the vet will probably ask is what you are feeding him on! Vets recognise the significance of diet to the animal's health but somewhere in the medical doctor's training the connection between diet and the human's health has been totally lost!

Drugs that are commonly dished out by doctors are constantly being blamed for increasing ill health. No testing is done on these drugs to ascertain what effect constant, daily poisoning with these unnatural compounds will have on an already sick person, over (sometimes) years. It would be unethical to use humans for such experimental testing, but that virtually is what is happening!

We all know about the Thalidomide scandal that rocked the pharmaceutical industry in the sixties. Now more and more drugs are proving to be dangerous to the human system with the cumulative effect of many years' prescribing by the well-meaning family doctor.

It is estimated today – in 1994 – that over *one million* patients are in hospital beds in the U.K. as a result of iatrogenesis (damaged caused by prescribed drugs)! (Source: *Journal of Alternative and Complementary Medicine;*

July 1994; article by Dr. Vernon Coleman, p28). The number of such admissions to hospitals in the U.S. must be many times more.

Professor Arnold Ehret states in his delightful little book *Rational Fasting* that when his patients are put on cleansing diets of fruits only, and the body starts aggressive elimination of stored toxins, he sees patients eliminate drugs they had taken as long as forty years before!

Instead of the prescribed-drug culture prevalent today, attention should be paid to the vast body of evidence that correct, natural diet can often reach the very cause and completely *cure* the condition.

Eminent doctors and scientists around the world, becoming increasingly disillusioned with drugs and their toxic side effects, are applying nutritional therapies to their patients. These scientists include the only double Nobel Prize Winner in history, the late Linus Pauling, who was awarded 40 honorary degrees from colleges and universities in the United States.

The application of proper nutrition influences positively the body's own healing mechanism, which we all have. The degree or speed of healing can vary from person to person. We all know of someone who seems to take longer to heal than the rest of us. Your doctor may put some iodine on a cut in your finger and cover it with a plaster. In due course the cut will heal, but it was not the doctor who did the healing. Your own body did the repair work.

If you break your leg, the doctor again may come to your aid and put a splint on the limb, and in time the broken bone will knit together, repairing itself. Again, it was not the doctor who healed the broken bone, it was your own body, your body's own healing power.

This innate intelligence that exists within your body is a supreme repairer of your bones and tissues.

This healing power does not just stop at broken bones and cuts, although we may just recognise these because they are the ones that most of us witness. Given the correct conditions, this healing power can correct all pathological conditions of the body, including cancer;

the Gerson Therapy is famous for achieving total remissions in very many terminal cancer cases who had been abandoned as hopeless by orthodox hospitals.

If our skin, or indeed any part of the body, develops a symptom, it is because that part is not receiving sufficient nutrition. If that part WERE to be supplied with the full quota of nutrients it requires for healthy functioning, then the condition would correct itself. In allergic reactions, the blood vessels supplying the reacting part of the body are interfered with, and the bloodflow in that area is stemmed, creating a deficiency symptom IN THAT AREA.

In disorders that are non-allergic in origin, restoration of the health of the patient is achievable by dietary improvement to 'kick-start' the innate healing power we all have.

Little is known about this invisible repair workshop. Its abilities are there to be witnessed, but the process itself remains a mystery. What I do know however, is that this supreme healing power actually requires correct nutrition to enable it to perform its undeniable miracles.

How do I know that for sure? Logical deduction really: if someone has deficiency symptoms, say spongy and bleeding gums (well-known vitamin C deficiency symptoms) and large doses of Vitamin C were supplied to the patient, the spongy and bleeding gums condition would correct itself.

If you were to watch that healing take place, you could rightly claim that you were witnessing this invisible healing power. Yet all it was, was a nutritional deficiency being corrected! But without that Vitamin C, that invisible healing power would not have functioned. It needed that Vitamin C to perform. Therefore this wonderful, 'invisible' healing power, must function properly under correct nutritionally-met conditions.

Conversely, if the vitamins and minerals are NOT there, this wonderful healing power would not work efficiently. Witness the slow healing power of wounds, when, again, Vitamin C is under supplied. That again is evidence that this healing power will function most sweetly when supplied with the correct nutrition.

When nutritional deficiencies persist and this deficiency state is aggravated over many years, this healing power can be further weakened, and whilst it may be able to carry out the repair of small cuts at a slow, but reasonably acceptable rate, the more demanding task of turning around a virulent cancer deep within the body may be beyond it – as evidenced by the number of people who indeed DO die from cancer.

However, by the same token, the number of people who have had virulent cancerous growths and who have been sent home to die, but have been restored to total health by such dietary therapies as the Gerson Therapy, is proof that by supplying the correct nutrition to the tissues in an intensive fashion to correct a deep deficiency state, the body's healing power can be restored, and the cancer defeated. In these cases, where nutrition fights and beats the cancer, an absolutely astonishing piece of physiological magic goes on in the body.

Beata Bishop recounts in *A Time to Heal*[66] after she had been on the Gerson Therapy for approximately 18 months, she realised there was a lump in her groin which, naturally, greatly worried her. It was decided to operate to remove the lump and have a pathologist report on it.

Much to her surprise, it turned out that her tumour had indeed been isolated, out of harm's way within the body, and the live tumour had shrunk and was enclosed in a *fifteen millimetre* thick capsule! The healing power, in its incredible wisdom had not only arrested the further spread of the disease, but had cornered the very nucleus of the tumour and walled it off so that it might do no more harm! To quote Beata Bishop on discovering the thickness of the encapsulation of the tumour: 'Fifteen? That's almost bulletproof!'

As it was, the lump was then surgically removed, purely as a precaution. But the lump itself told its own story, inasmuch as it was evident that the cancer was, to all intents and purposes, 'outwith' the body. It had been encased in a calcified cocoon, out of harm's way. It had been defeated, and well and truly trapped.

But what if she had not had it surgically removed, but had left it in her body? Because the live cancerous cells in the very heart of the encapsulation were also surrounded by dead cells, one can hypothesise that these live cells were on borrowed time and would eventually have met with the same fate as the dead cells surrounding them and that slowly they too would have died off.

And the likely scenario after that would have been for the entire 'lump' to have slowly dissolved and been removed from the body (as in the *The Grape Cure*, a book written by Basil Shackleton who relates that, after six weeks on nothing but grapes and water, his tumour was dissolved by the healing power of the fruit and carried out of his body in his urine; he had the excreted mass confirmed by a London pathologist as being the dissolved tumour).

The above happened to Beata because her healing power – which is no different from yours or mine – had been supplied with the correct nutrition, so that it could work at its greatest efficiency. It obviously had not been working efficiently in the first place or she would not have originally incurred the cancer.

And in another documented case of recovery from cancer (Case No. 23, *A Cancer Therapy by Max Gerson M.D. pp325–329*), a 43 year old lady who had a malignant tumour in her left thigh had a fracture repaired by the insertion of strong, metal screws.

In healing on the therapy, the power of the new growing bone tissue was so great that it broke four screws into pieces!

Such fascinating occurrences as detailed above never cease to amaze me when I hear of them. That encapsulation of a tumour, miraculous though it may sound, is apparently quite normal when dietary therapies are applied to cancers.

Such a dietary treatment for cancer is today widely recognised by the Dutch government and is widely available in hospitals throughout Holland. The Moerman Diet was 'invented' by a Dutch G.P. by the name of Cornelis Moerman, who, in the 1930s – after Gerson discovered his dietary treatment – arrived at his own dietary treatment for cancer. His and Gerson's diets are very similar, but in my opinion the Gerson version is far more efficacious and successful.

In a book written by a writer, Ruth Jochems, called the *Moerman Cancer Diet*, the actual process of encapsulating a tumour seems well established and nothing at all out of the ordinary! To quote from the publication:

'Dr. Moerman's natural cure divides the healing process into three stages:

1.   Stopping the growth of the tumour.
2.   Walling off the tumour by encapsulation.
3.   Breaking the tumour down.

To make the method work the patient needs three things:

1.   The diet.
2.   The vitamin supplements.
3.   A will of iron.

If you've got all three, you can cure yourself!'

So the fascinating encapsulating of a tumour, which would probably make the eyes of a 'normal' cancer doctor stand out on stalks, is a well-recognised phenomenon, and it seems to be expected no matter where the dietary therapy is applied.

Whether it's the Moerman diet in Holland or, many thousands of miles away, the Gerson Therapy in Mexico. A mere half-a-world apart changes nothing; the process is the same. This is simply because the elements that are involved – man and nutrients – are the same, no matter where in the world you go.

As in all the other cases of healing through dietary treatment, in each successful case the body's own healing power has responded positively with the renewed and vigorous application of super-nutrition to the system. Without the proper nutrition the healing power is hampered and if over-tasked will become ineffectual. But restore correct nutrition to the body and all manner of little symptoms, as well as all manner of serious disorders, may disappear. The huge number of success stories in Nature Cure history (and I include the Gerson Therapy in this category), bears witness to the ability of the healing power to be re-activated in order to combat effectively, all manner of diseases.

But if you are ill, merely eating the correct foods may not in itself be enough to restore this amazing inbuilt healing power. The nutritional components have to be able to be absorbed and properly assimilated, and the mere fact that you are ill in the first place may well indicate a weakened ability to use the very foods that can help you. Therefore, as in the Gerson, the taking of digestive enzymes to assist the absorption is essential. It can be that you may get well without these enzymes, but it will take much longer as slowly, bit by bit, the nutrition leaks through and equally slowly restores digestion function, which in turn helps further (but still very slowly) the digestion and absorption of the next incoming nutrients. This can take many months, whereas with the enzymes, the progress can be accelerated.

The Gerson Therapy

The story of the Gerson Therapy is a wonderful, inspiring one, and at the same time extremely sad because of the way its discoverer was treated by the medical profession in America.

Max Gerson M.D., was born in Germany in 1881. A migraine sufferer, he was told by his doctor that he would have to live with it. Undeterred, Gerson, after reading of an Italian doctor who had successfully controlled his own migraine by diet, experimented with his own and found that, by eliminating some foods and eating raw fruits and vegetables, his migraine disappeared.

He later applied the dietary principles that he had learned, with great success to his own migraine patients.

One day, one of his migraine sufferers reported to Dr. Gerson that his lupus vulgaris – or skin T.B. – was going away. Dr. Gerson expressed disbelief because everyone knew that lupus was an 'incurable' disease. But the evidence was there before his eyes – the lupus was indeed healing! Dr. Gerson reasoned – rightly, it turned out

– that the body, on this natural-food diet, was healing itself. Other lupus patients soon came to him. They too, were cured. Gerson found that patients with secondary complaints such as arthritis and other so-called incurable illnesses, had these afflictions similarly helped by the diet.

Gerson's treatment soon reached the ears of a Professor Sauerbruch in Austria – a world-famous thoracic surgeon and tuberculosis authority. He showed great interest in Gerson's claims to cure lupus and invited a trial with lupus patients at his Austrian clinic.

It transpired that Sauerbruch's clinical trial of Gerson's dietary treatment proved an astonishing success, with lasting cures in 446 out of 450 lupus sufferers! (This event is related in Sauerbruch's own autobiography: *Master Surgeon*.)

Instead of being awarded the Nobel Prize as might have been expected, Gerson was called before a court, by irritated and doubtless embarrassed physicians, to defend his treatment. Gerson won his case but this resistance by orthodox medicine against a successful dietary treatment was to prove an on-going feature for the rest of his life.

When he fled to America to avoid Hitler's hounding of the Jews, his diet had now become successful in curing very many terminally ill cancer patients. And he had the biopsies performed by outside hospitals so that he could not be accused of fiddling his records. X-rays taken before and after treatment, showing tumours gone, were available to all visiting physicians. Gerson was so keen to share his success that he invited the American Medical Association down to his clinic.

They came, saw all his records, and left without saying much. Despite all Gerson's marvellous success stories with extremely difficult terminal patients who had been sent home to die and had now fully recovered under Gerson's treatment, the AMA labelled him under the 'Frauds and Fables' category!

You have to understand that the hugely-powerful Pharmaceutical giants funded the medical schools, who in turn taught their doctors to prescribe drugs, drugs and more drugs, forever boosting the drug industries' profits. If Gerson's simple dietary treatment were to be accepted, these massive corporations would be practically wiped out. There is no money in dietary treatment, except for the greengrocer, Gerson often remarked.

It was made a crime in California to treat cancer by this non-toxic approach and instead the authorities insisted on extremely toxic and dangerous chemotherapy and radiation, which, according to the Gerson Institute, had a zero-percent success rate.

Some medical doctors, who had developed cancer themselves and cured themselves by Gerson's dietary approach, would not treat their own cancer patients this way for fear of losing their licence.

The Gerson Institute is still going strong today, but they had to take their clinic over the border to Mexico where they are much more tolerant of 'alternative' therapies.

In Gerson's experience, no matter where about in the body a tumour may exist, and if the patient went to Gerson at not too late a stage, the very same diet was able to 'access' the growth and deal with it. Whether it be in the head, or the leg, the identical diet was able to restore health to the entire body, which included the site of the tumour.

But what is commonplace on the Gerson diet is the fact that people with cancers may have secondary health complaints and, whilst on the diet, these too clear up. One such patient, who suffered from syphillis, saw the condition totally clear up without any need for anti-syphillitic drugs. Diabetes too, is a disorder which responds well with the regimen and patients sooner or later dispense with their insulin medication.

The fact that the one diet can, in so many different people, restore health no matter where in the body the disorder may be, is ample proof that the fabulous healing power we all have within us, applies its abilities to the body as a whole and is not selective, i.e. it will not just repair one part of the body and leave the rest alone; it will seek out all disorders, and, if the vitality of that human is not too badly compromised, restore total health to that area.

Gerson detailed his dietary therapy, along with 50 full case histories complete with X-rays, in his book, *A Cancer Therapy. Results of Fifty Cases.*

The highly-intensive Gerson Therapy comprises a non-toxic diet of 13 freshly pressed raw vegetable and fruit juices per day as well as a saltless, largely raw, diet of fresh fruits and vegetables with some (non-toxic) medications.

Why Don't Doctors Know About Diet as a Means of Healing?

Probably THE most important question affecting the health of everybody in the entire civilised world today!

Doctors lose sight of the fact that when healthy, primitive, peoples are introduced to Western processed diets – the Samoans and the Hunzas are only two examples – they develop our Western diseases.

To quote from *Nutrition and Physical Degeneration* by Weston A. Price D.D.S., who travelled the world comparing the healths of primitive civilisations:

'If any one impression of our experiences were to be selected as particularly vivid, it would be the contrast between the health and ruggedness of the primitives in general and that of the foreigners who have entered their country. That their superior ruggedness was not racial became evident when through contact with modern civilization's degenerative processes developed.'

There are many reasons for doctors not accepting the concept; some appalling.

Firstly, and most importantly, doctors don't know about it! As simple as that. Doctors are not taught it at medical school so they cannot be expected to know. They are taught to diagnose symptoms, label the condition, and supply drugs which hopefully will influence the patient's disorder to the good.

Why they are NOT taught about restoration of health by dietary means, leaves more questions unanswered than answered.

If dietary treatments were to become the norm, the massive pharmaceutical giants would be financially crippled. In America, according to information available, the medical schools are funded by these multi-billion dollar corporations, to encourage them to teach doctors to dispense drugs, forever boosting their profits. I am unclear of the situation in Britain, but I have read many informed articles wherein it has been suggested that doctors are, to all intents and purposes, in the pockets of the massively-wealthy drug companies.

Couple the fact that doctors are not trained in nutrition – and not simply nutrition – but the absolute link between correct diet and the body's healing ability, with the massively persuasive drug and profit-oriented machinery of the giant drug companies and you can readily see why the pharmaceutical companies would like not one bit for the dietary approach to ill-health to see the light of day.

That 'nature cure' works is beyond question. It may not work in 100 out of 100 cases, but it has had results with all sorts of conditions, that to anybody's eyes would be described as 'miraculous'. However, it is slow – like all of nature's physiological processes; getting fat and losing weight are two fine examples – often depressingly slow – and overwhelmingly unpopular, because of the widespread processed-food addictions that all Westernised populations now have.

The story of the Hunzas, which resulted from extensive laboratory experiments by none other than the eminent English surgeon, Sir Robert McCarrison, proved beyond a shadow of a doubt that the supreme health of these primitive people was down entirely to their diet. He spent seven years amongst them and did not see one solitary case of our commonplace Western degenerative diseases.

When he fed laboratory rats on the Hunza diet, they became well-grown, with sleek shiny fur, strong and playful with each other, and long lived. Another group of laboratory rats – kept in identical conditions so as not to confuse the outcome – were fed the civilised 'English' diet, and they developed poor fur, had little energy and fought with each other, indicating they were miserable. They also did not live long. Furthermore, and probably more telling, was the fact McCarrison would take diseased and ill rats, put them on the Hunza diet – AND THEY GOT WELL!

The same happened with Pottenger who experimented with huge colonies of cats. The results were identical.

Gerson has recorded results second to none in the world, of fully recovered, formerly terminally ill, cancer patients.

Orthodox medical practitioners, after training for five years without the slightest instruction in Nature Cure are understandably nonplussed when asked by their patients, who know more about this subject than their doctor, why they don't use diet as a means of restoring health.

Doctors applaud you if you tell them you are changing to a healthy diet. But if you tell them that the REASON you are changing it, is to treat any illness you may have, then they do not like that one little bit!

Firstly, they are embarrassed because they don't know the subject. Secondly, it seems awfully simple! In this day of high technology, surely the answer to all illness – they consider – lies in the 21st century laboratory. Thirdly, they feel threatened. How would you feel after training for five years or so, to find out you've been barking up the wrong tree? I do not think you would want to know that. And that's exactly the sort of attitude you will more often than not get if you show the average doctor a book on curing by diet.

One has seriously got to pose the question: If testing in laboratories with animals is good enough to give doctors and pharmaceutical companies sufficient evidence to prove the efficacy of any number of drugs and treatments, why then cannot they recognise the outcome of other animal experiments? Namely:

> *The animal experiments by Sir Robert McCarrison*
> *and*
> *The animal experiments by Francis Pottenger M.D.*

Besides the above fascinating experiments which prove that dietary means of healing are actually far SUPERIOR to 'orthodox medicine', especially for serious diseases, there is abundant evidence from the Gerson Institute, which includes full case histories, X-rays, biopsy results etc., which confirm the findings of McCarrison and Pottenger.

Before the reader arrives at the opinion that I am against orthodox medicine, I should point out that every one of my heroes is a doctor: Gerson, McCarrison, Pottenger, amongst others. However I'll admit to having little time for those of the profession who cannot see beyond the training that they received at medical school.

THIRTEEN

Other Dietary Myths

All readers of this book will probably accept that fruits and vegetables are the foods we SHOULD eat, and that it is our over-indulgence in other foods that is causing the widespread health disorders in our industrialised societies.

The primitive Hunzakuts, about whom we shall read further on, had no such health problems as cancer, heart disease, and all the other 'civilised' illnesses. Further, the eminent surgeon, Sir Robert McCarrison *proved* that their freedom from disease was due to their diet, and their diet alone.

We, in the 'West' are so programmed into thinking that the foods on supermarket shelves constitute 'normal food' that we lose sight of the fact that it is these very tinned and processed foods – so different from the food Nature intended us to eat – that are largely responsible for our many health problems.

We nearly all eat from supermarkets, or at least eat the products which are regularly on offer there. These foods are nearly always interfered with in the name of profit; they are practically all denatured.

Food processors and manufacturers are in existence to make money and if they can find a way of producing something that doesn't spoil quickly – extend its shelf life in the shops – they will do it. To that end nearly everything in the supermarket has been heated and practically everything that is tinned is 'dead' food. Even the supermarket's 'natural' produce of fruits and vegetables will almost certainly have been interfered with by commercial tactics to prevent their destruction whilst growing in the field (pesticides and other insect repellant sprays). No person on this planet knows what long-term, cumulative effect the regular consumption of such toxic chemicals will have on man, but commonsense dictates that such daily poisoning can only lead to health problems, sooner or later!

The corn flakes on the supermarket shelf are a million miles removed from the natural corn which once grew in the field. It will almost certainly have been heated, roasted, toasted, shaped, pressurized and all manner of interference bestowed upon it; all for the purpose of increasing its appeal. This manipulation of a previously-natural foodstuff robs it of many nutrients and, in an attempt to appeal to the health-conscious consumer, the manufacturers guiltily add in some meagre amounts of synthetic vitamins hoping that will impress the head of the household.

Fresh foods are rich in vitamins, minerals, enzymes, co-enzymes and many other nutrients that have not yet been isolated or 'discovered' by food scientists; the yet-to-be-discovered nutrients. These nutrients, although not identified, are, and always have been, in natural, untampered foods. No manufacturer of processed foods can replace those nutritional elements which were put there by nature for a purpose.

As you eat, over many years, these dead, over-heated and processed 'foods', which are lacking in the very enzymes which would accompany them in nature for their use and assimilation within the body, the waste products of these foods are not eliminated as efficiently as they should be and these deposits build up, clogging the human system and in turn causing health problems.

The human body is little more than a collection of pipes and tubes and it is when these get clogged up that health problems surface. The circulation of the blood is inter-fered with and all manner of disorders − dependent where about in the body the 'clogging' takes place − will arise. Heart attacks and blood clots are typical examples of major obstructions but lesser blood vessels can have the circulation to them reduced or interfered with by such clogging and symptoms will then inevitably surface.

One very famous naturopath, Professor Arnold Ehret, a former professor at Baden Baden in Germany, who cured himself of a terminal illness (Bright's disease) by changing to a fruit only diet, stated that the body is like a watch and an ill body is like a dirty watch that is clogged up and simply needs cleaning!

To clean out your body you need fruits and green leafy vegetables! It may sound a recipe for boredom and it probably is, because all our Westernised tastes are perverted and many of us would turn our noses up at such 'rabbit food'. But it is the food that man lived solely on many thousands of years ago. We in the West have never been so unhealthy as we are today. The U.K. and the U.S.A. have seen increasing poor health amongst their populations for decades: It is getting far worse, not better!

And don't believe it when you are told that we are living longer: We're not! The Queen may be sending out more and more 100-year-old birthday telegrams in the U.K. each year but the reason that is, is because people have to *ask* for one to be sent and it is the growing number of people who are only now aware of that fact that distorts the true picture! Look around any old graveyard and you will see ample evidence of long-lived people. Many died younger centuries ago simply because of bad sanitation and these many infant deaths played a part in distorting the *average* lifespan of these times!

There is hope however, for all of you who think that you could never survive on such healthy foods as fruits and vegetables; your taste changes! After only a few days on fruits only, you can actually start to relish the prospect of some sweet grapes, or luscious ripe tomatoes; Believe me – it is quite true!

If you were to go on such a health-building regimen as fruits and vegetables only, you will doubtless be discouraged from doing so by well-meaning people around you – relatives and friends – who will think you are on a dangerous diet! It is THEY who are digging their graves with their teeth, whilst you will be cleansing old toxins out

of your body and travelling down on the road to supreme
health, free from allergies, weight problems and all the
other health disorders commonly seen around us.

You will however encounter people who will suggest
you are not getting enough protein by eating simply fruits
and vegetables. This, and the other buzz-word of today,
cholesterol, will now be dealt with.

The Protein Myth

Most modern-day dieticians believe that each one of us
has to have protein every day – from an animal source.
Or else we will have serious protein deficiencies.

But this protein myth, like so much spurious information
in nutrition, has not been thought out too clearly by those
animal-protein advocates.

Although 'protein' deficiencies can occur in barren parts
of Africa, for example, it is not just protein that creates
the kwashiorkor syndrome, but the lack of food including
protein! Protein through a natural diet of fruits and vegetables (which contain vegetable proteins) and some nuts
or seeds, is quite sufficient for the human system to
thrive on.

It is thought that man has to eat animal meat in order
to get protein; that you have to eat meat to grow muscle
– that is the theory. The scientists reckon that muscle,
tissues, and the entire body's essential substance is
protein, therefore this substance must be eaten in order
to build and to grow more protein. You must eat muscle
to build muscle, you must eat protein to build protein,
you must eat fat to build fat, and in the case of a nursing
mother, she must drink milk to make milk!

The cow builds its flesh, tissues, bones, hair, milk, efficiency, energy, and heat, all from *grass* exclusively! Yet we
eat the cow thinking we need the cow's meat to build our
own muscle – our own protein. Some scientists think that
we cannot build muscles from fruits and vegetables.

If a farmer were to feed milk to a cow to increase
milk production, other farmers would think he was
mad. Yet our food scientists often tell us the nursing

mother has to drink milk in order for her body to make milk.

It is true that eskimos eat nothing but meat and that they are healthy. But they too are exactly adhering to the requirements of Nature; eating untampered foods – fresh and raw! Man is omnivorous; he can eat fruits, vegetables and meat, but for people who have health or weight problems, then a fruit and vegetable diet is the number one diet for restoring health. Remember too, that only a small part of the world (the Arctic and Antarctic) was 'made' without plant life, so fruits and vegetables should be the first choice of food for man, who was given canine teeth specifically so that, should the need arise, he would have the ability to survive in such cold, plantless climes.

The Different Views

Authorities in different countries are divided over the amount of protein each of us should eat per day. At the turn of the century the respected authorities were Rubner and Volt, who said we needed 120–160 grams per day. Chittenden then showed in human experiments that best performance and health were assured on 50 grams. Hinhede set the figure at 30 gms. Today, decades and much protein research later, the situation is no different. There is still much confusion. In Russia Jakovlev set up a minimum requirement of 144–163 grams. Kuhnau put the optimum at 200. Kofranyi of the Max Planck Institute proved that complete health could be maintained on a mere 25 grams! Then Oomen and Hipsley found a population that develop robust health on a mere 15 grams, with magnificent muscular structure and excellent physical performance!

The textbooks say that vegetable protein is inferior to animal protein. Yet there have been populations numbering in the millions in various parts of the earth who are known, from penetrating research, to have developed enviable health and strength for thousands of years on a purely vegetarian diet. McCollum, the discoverer of vitamin D, showed in 1923 the high protein quality of a whole wheat and green vegetable combination. Abelin reported the same results in 1942 in the Swiss Medical Journal. According to Verzar in 1956, ten different purely vegetable protein combinations of the highest biological quality were known to the Food and Agriculture Organisation of the UN. About 20 years ago it was shown at the Max Planck Institute for Nutritional Physiology that the previous bases for calculation, which had shown animal protein to be essential, were erroneous![67]

Another point needed to be made on the protein myth; the ape is considered to be the closest animal, physiologically and anatomically-speaking, to man. Look at the muscular development of the ape; the huge frame, the massive strength. The scientists obviously have not thought too clearly on that one. This mountain of an animal, so closely related, even in bodily organ distribution and functions, eats no meat, but exists extremely healthily in the wild on fruits and plant foods. Another giant of a beast over-endowed with muscular strength is the elephant, another is the rhinoceros. Neither of them is protein deficient, or a weakling, yet their strength and their protein comes directly from plant foods.

The Cholesterol Myth

Newspapers and books are full of advice, as are indeed doctors, to cut to down on the fats you eat or else you will end up with clogging of the arteries (arteriosclerosis). Often these are the same people who will refute any connection between diet and health . . .

But there is a ton of evidence to suggest that cholesterol in a diet does *not* produce arteriosclerosis.

The word 'Eskimo' is derived from an American Indian language, and means 'he who eats it raw'. The primitive Eskimo has no access to plant foods and eats most of his high-meat diet raw. They eat much fat and meat and they do NOT get arteriosclerosis and they are a hardy and healthy race. W.O. Douglas wrote in May 1964, in the *National Geographic*: 'The Banks Island Eskimos said that frozen fish and frozen caribou seem to provide more "strength" than cooked food.'

K. Birket-Smith in his book *The Eskimo* noted that meat is stored to undergo autolysis, which produces new flavours, so that 'walrus meat tastes like old, sharp and rich cheese.' In C.M. Garber's Eating with the Eskimos[68] he said: 'Alaskan Eskimos are heavy eaters of lean meats and large amounts of blubber. In only a few instances did they cook their food. The usual and customary method was to devour it raw.' He noted that the Eskimos thrive on titmuck, which is frozen, raw fish, reduced to a consistency requiring it to be ladled.

The anthropologist V. Stefansson lived among the Eskimos of northern Canada for 7 years and became an authority on primitive Eskimo life. His reports appeared in many journals where he emphasised the excellent state of their health and freedom from disease.

Cholesterol is essential to our bodies. It makes up a large part of our brain and cell membranes. Production of our adrenal and sex hormones and of vitamin D depend on cholesterol. But, as you do not need to eat protein to create protein within our bodies, so too can our bodies make cholesterol out of practically *any* food that we eat. We do NOT need to eat cholesterol to make cholesterol within our bodies. The immediate biochemical precursor of our cholesterol is the compound Acetyl Coenzyme A, which is a common point in the metabolism of proteins, fats, and carbohydrates. Thus, any food can lead to cholesterol manufacture.[69]

Therefore, the common belief that eating a diet high in cholesterol creates heart disease, is quite wrong. True, high cholesterol levels are indicative of a likelihood of developing coronary heart disease. But it hasn't been proven that lowering individual lipid levels in any way prevents heart disease.[70]

In fact, Dr. Ian Macdonald of Guy's Hospital in London has been able to show that serum lipids can be influenced by the amount of dietary *carbohydrate* you eat.[71]

It appears high blood cholesterol levels are caused not by eating eggs or fats but by poor nutrition. Correcting the diet to a natural, unrefined one will lower these levels.

Dr. Edward Howell in Enzyme Nutrition[72] suggests

that faulty fatty metabolism can be the cause for the body's poor handling of cholesterol in the diet.

But the most convincing parallel to my mind is a 'Research Contribution' by Maynard Murray M.D. (also in Enzyme Nutrition). Dr. Howell's introduction remarks that Dr. Murray relates how he participated in anatomical dissection of whales and seals, unearthing the astounding and challenging revelation that their arteries were healthy and free from cholesterol, in spite of the fact that their harsh environment requires consumption of fat without restraint! These warm-blooded animals seem to eat large amounts of fat with impunity. Whales and seals need a heavy layer of insulating fat under the skin to keep warm and should be prime candidates for atherosclerosis, but they have none! This was Dr. Maynard Murray's observation:

'Fat in Whales and Seals

Within the years 1942–1945, under the auspices of Archer, Daniels, Midland Company of Chicago, between 900–1000 sperm whales were dissected in Peru. The only pathology sought in these animals involved malignancies, arteriosclerosis, and arthritis. None of these were found. We also measured the size of the thymus gland which persisted in these animals; weight 80 to 100 pounds in the slaughtered carcass. While microscopic sections of these glands were not numerous, however, the tissue examined showed them to be active and not replaced by fat or fibrous tissue. The coronary arteries microscopically did not show any atherosclerosis; neither did the aortas. There was approximately 8 inches of saturated subcutaneous fat in whales, yet no hardening of the arteries.

Off the Aleutian Islands of Alaska, around 3,000 seals were dissected after being slaughtered for their fur. No malignant tumours were found, and there was no pathology in their arteries and joints. We dissected about 30 small Harp Seals which were slaughtered on ice floes off the eastern coast of Canada. These animals also showed no pathology of the kinds mentioned above.'

I think the message therefore is quite clear: Obey nature's rules and do not interfere with her intended foods — eat naturally – and ill health will be avoided. The foods (meats) the Eskimos ate would be untampered with: As nature intended. The meat would be eaten on its own, for maximum utilisation by the body; there would be no mixed plates of protein and starches.

The meat would not be pumped full of antibiotics or growth hormones or other substances in an effort to make the animal bigger, and therefore more profitable for the supplier. The poor Westernised man eats not only meat which has been tampered with but all sorts of deficient, refined foods which, all added together, make for a deficient, unnatural diet, that creates all sorts of havoc within the body. And Dr. Howell's faulty fatty metabolism theory seems highly plausible, especially in view of the offerings in this book that food allergies themselves can interfere with the body's metabolism and so result in obesity (which, in turn, leads to illhealth).

The Hunzas: A Nutritional Lesson for us All

Perhaps the most famous example of excellence in the health of man must be the Hunza people, or properly referred to as the Hunzakuts, who live in a remote part of the Himalayas.

When Sir Robert McCarrison, an eminent English surgeon visited this remote tribespeople in the 1920s, he came back full of stories of the fabulous health and physiques that were constant throughout their remote community. Where they lived was so cut off from the outside that they had to be self-sufficient in all that they did – and ate.

McCarrison had never seen a people who were so completely free of all disease and ill health. They lived very long and active lives, with the men fathering children in their 90s and anyone of 80 was considered middle-aged!

After extensive research and experiments, McCarrison was able to prove conclusively that their supreme health, vitality and freedom from disease was no mere fluke but was totally due to their natural diet. Furthermore, by feeding diseased rats the Hunza diet, their healths were restored; further proof if proof be needed that the number one factor in health is, and always will be, diet.

The supremely-healthy Hunza diet[73] consisted of leafy green vegetables, fruits – chiefly apricots and mulberries – fresh and sun-dried, wholegrains, potatoes and other root vegetables; peas and beans, gram of chick pea and other pulses, fresh, raw milk and buttermilk, or lassi, and meat only on very rare occasions. They drank water from the mountain glaciers.

It is a sad reflection on what might be considered 'progress' that the Hunza people – now accessible to outsiders and indulging in their visitors' foods – are now starting to show signs of illhealth that mirror our own industrialised nations' horrific catalogue of modern diseases.

FOURTEEN

The Yet-to-be-Discovered Nutrients

It wasn't so long ago that vitamins were discovered. One by one their presence was noted by scientists. Soon after each was discovered, so too was its deficiency state observed.

With each one came a new insight into human health. Each time it was thought that that one substance might just be the answer to all our prayers. And so it went on; through vitamin A, onto the B vitamins, and then through the other letters. Each time, new hope blossomed. Was *this* finally our secret to long life and happiness? Each time a nutrient was isolated, another flurry of scientific activity emerged, with books written about the pros and cons of each of these seemingly miraculous but tiny chemical substances.

Then the minerals were 'discovered'. Each one again creating waves of excitement in the scientific and health world. More books on each and every one of these substances appeared. Many proclaiming that deficiencies or excesses of these inorganic chemical substances would solve or create this or that health problem.

Then it was the turn of the amino acids – all 22 of them – and each one had its claim to fame. Next came the enzymes. The number of enzymes permutated from amino acid chains is innumerable. In 1947 there were 200 known enzymes.[74] In 1957, 660. In 1962 there were 850; and by 1968 science had identified 1300 of them! If you wanted to find out how many enzymes are known today, you would need to hire specialist scientists full time to survey the many thousands that have been found!

All the claims for these enzymes add to the plethora of information daily being processed by science. And rightly so. Any nutritional discovery is a step forward. Any improvement of knowledge on the link between our health and our diet should be applauded and welcomed.

But these substances, although 'discovered' only this century, have been in existence since Adam bit into his first Granny Smith's. These substances -- along with the ones which will be 'discovered' years from now – have been taken into the bodies of us humans ever since the world began. The enzymes that will be discovered in the year 2050 were in existence in the bodies of George Washington and Marco Polo. So they're not new!

These substances have been focused on with enormous scientific muscle, and there will certainly be many more discoveries – that is guaranteed.

You can bet your bottom dollar that when these new nutrients are found it will be shown that a deficiency of the new nutrient causes so-and-so symptoms and/or a toxic amount will create other signs of illhealth.

But remember, as we can be eating these undiscovered nutrients now – this very day – so, too, can we be deficient in them if we are not eating natural foods, our only source of them. So, at this very moment, you might be suffering from the deficiency symptoms of the yet-to-be-discovered Nutrient X, but because no one has found Nutrient X, or worked out its deficiency symptoms, your health problems will, for the moment, sit in the box labelled 'of psychosomatic origin' or 'of unknown aetiology'!

Which reminds me of a doctor's quote many years ago. I have forgotten his name, so cannot honour him with its origin. But he said 'When a doctor says a symptom is psychosomatic, that is just another way of saying he doesn't know what's wrong with you.' It's a convenient get-out in other words.

So, all the illhealth that abounds in our doctors' surgeries may well be the deficiency states of nutrients still to be discovered. It would certainly explain something very well known by natural healers; that by correcting the patient's diet to a natural one, their health slowly – but surely – returns. Isn't this just the sort of thing that would happen in the correction of a nutrient deficiency?

Do not forget, also, that diseases can be the result of combinations of deficiencies,[75] so if you take all the known nutrients and note their KNOWN deficiencies and then add all the possible UNKNOWN nutrients along with their unknown deficiency symptoms, the possible deficiency symptoms caused by combining them in all sorts of permutations are mind-boggling! And too, the possible combination-remedies, with the right balances, is an impossible task to even consider working out.

Scientists can keep on focusing on isolated parts of the body, or single nutrients, or parts of organs and tissue. They can keep discovering new vitamins and other nutrients and witness the accompanying euphoria. They can keep discovering new liaisons between connective tissues or brain fibres. They can keep on learning about the behaviour of neurotransmitters within the brain. They can keep discovering how something works, which they might not have known before. But I think it should be clear to the reader, that overall, the answer which will accommodate ALL of these discoveries and ALL of the ones yet to be discovered in the future, has been with man from the beginning of the world: natural, untampered food.

Nutrients and their Deficiency States

The commonest nutrients are listed below. It should go without saying that all these nutrients should come from fresh fruits, vegetables etc., within our actual diets, but with our modern, processed foods, these nutrients are often reduced or even missing, so be aware that such deficient diets can cause many disorders.

Vitamin A

Deficiency: night blindness, xerophthalmia (dryness/ulceration of cornea).

Carotene, a substance in yellow and green vegetables and fruits that changes into Vitamin A, is not well absorbed unless textures are unusually soft. Thus many individuals obtain too little Vitamin A unless their diets are supplemented. It has been known for centuries that there is a substance in liver, beneficial in certain eye diseases. It was named vitamin A in 1917 by McCollum and Simmonds. Vitamin A can be toxic, but an adult would have to have taken 100,000 to 500,000 units daily for 15 months or longer before any symptoms became noticeable.[76,77,78,79]

Sources: cream, butter, whole milk, eggs, and liver.

Vitamin B1 (Thiamine)

Deficiency: Beriberi.
Beriberi occurs essentially where rice as the staple food is highly polished (the outer husks removed from the brown rice to make it look white and attractive). It is still an important public health problem in some countries of South and East Asia. Sub-clinical (not fullblown) symptoms can be: Lack of initiative, lack of appetite, depression, irritability, poor memory, tendency to tire easily and inability to concentrate. Vital to muscle coordination, it is an essential nutrient amongst men and women who drink a lot of alcohol. Deficiency has been known to mimic heart attacks in alcoholics. B1 has been used to treat hundreds of conditions.

Sources: wholegrain cereals, nuts, dairy produce, fruits, vegetables.

Vitamin B2 (Riboflavin)

Deficiency: cracking and inflammation at the edges of the lips, a reddened inflamed tongue, and bloodshot, burning, tearing and light-sensitive eyes are signs of B2 deficiency. Some studies link this vitamin with depression. Karrer and Kuhn successfully completed the synthesis of riboflavin in 1935.

Sources: yeast, milk, liver, lean meat, fish, cheese, eggs, green vegetables, and wholegrain cereals.

Vitamin B3 (Niacin)

Deficiency: Pellagra: loss of weight, anorexia, soreness of the tongue and mouth, indigestion, diarrhoea, insomnia and mental confusion.

A well known aid to memory recalls Pellagra as the disease of the 3 Ds: 'Dermatitis, diarrhoea and dementia'. Discovered by Huber in 1867, this vitamin has been used with considerable success in schizophrenia in the USA and Canada. The Nicotinic acid version of Niacin produces flushing of the skin, which can be frightening when experienced for the first time, but it is temporary. If you want to avoid the flushing, take the Amide form, either as nicotinamide or niacinamide.

Sources: wholegrain cereals, yeast, liver, poultry, legumes, fish, fruits, vegetables, dairy products.

B5 (Calcium pantothenate, or pantothenic Acid)

Deficiency: abdominal pain, nausea, sleeplessness, emotional upsets, weakness and cramps.

Discovered by nutritional scientist Professor Roger Williams of the University of Texas.

Sources: organ meats, vegetables, fish, wholegrain cereals, nuts, most food groups.

B6 (Pyridoxine)

Deficiency: inability to recall dreams. Nervousness, insomnia, abdominal pain, irritability, weakness and difficulty in walking. First synthesised in 1939 by Kuhn in Germany and by Harris and Folkers in the U.S.A.

Besides an inability to recall dreams, a test for deficiency is to bend your fingers so the tips touch where your fingers join your hand. If they don't touch, you may have a B6 deficiency. Women who are pregnant, and women on the Contraceptive Pill run the risk of deficiency. They are recommended to take 50 to 100 milligrams of pyridoxine daily (preferably in capsule form).

Sources: meats, liver, vegetables, whole grain cereals, egg yolk, most food groups.

B12 (Cyanocobalamin)

Deficiency: pernicious anaemia. Neuritis, poor growth, sore tongue.

In 1948 it was announced both by Lester Smith in England and Rickes in America that they had isolated the anti-pernicious anaemia factor in pure crystalline form.

Sources: animal protein foods.

Inositol

Deficiency: none as yet established.

First discovered as a food factor in 1850 but not recognised as a B vitamin until 1940.

Sources: fish, eggs, lecithin.

Choline

Deficiency: circulatory disease, such as high blood pressure or excess cholesterol may be due to choline deficiency.

Known to science as a food factor since 1849.

Sources: fish, eggs, lecithin.

Biotin

Deficiency: rare in adults. Babies may show anaemia, dermatitis, scaly skin and diarrhoea. Can be produced within the body, but antibiotics can create deficiency.

Discovered by Bateman in 1916 but synthesised by Harris and colleagues in the U.S.A. in 1948.

Sources: wholegrain cereals, seeds, nuts, vegetables, legumes, eggs and milk products.

PABA (Para-amino-benzoic-acid)

Deficiency: none yet established, but is effective sunscreen therefore perhaps involved in tanning mechanism.

PABA was first synthesised by Fischer in 1863 but only became a B vitamin in 1940.

Sources: wholegrain cereals, seeds, nuts, vegetables, beans, lentils, yeast, eggs and milk products.

Folic Acid (Folatin)

Deficiency: anaemia, weakness, fatigue, breathlessness and certain mental illness symptoms.

Discovered in 1941 by Mitchell, Snell and Williams.

Sources: wholegrain cereals, seeds, nuts, vegetables, beans, lentils, yeast, eggs and milk products.

Vitamin C

Deficiency: Scurvy. Symptoms: lack of energy, easy fatigue, aching in bones, joints and muscles especially at night, allergies, wrinkles, premature ageing, bleeding gums, dental cavities, easy bruising, nose bleeds, slow healing of wounds, anaemia.

Vitamin C is the most famous of all the vitamins. Vitamin C is known as Ascorbic Acid, but was originally called Hexuronic Acid. Funk 'discovered' Vitamin C in 1912, but it was isolated by Gyorgyi in 1928. It was Gyorgyi who named it Hexuronic Acid. The Vikings did not experience scurvy on long sea voyages; their safeguard was to carry on each ship a large barrel of apples! Jacques Cartier, in 1536, set out to explore the St. Lawrence River. He arrived with his entire crew sick and 26 men already dead from (what later became known as) scurvy. He put ashore several of his desperately ill men to die as there was nothing further he could do. A few days later the captain, when he went ashore, found his men miraculously cured. The Indians had given them a tea made with the young green shoots (the needles) of the spruce tree.

In 1747, James Lind, a Scottish naval surgeon, conducted experiments with different diets on his crew who had become ill with this dreaded disease. One of these diets included oranges and lemons. These men were restored to health within a few days! Later it became compulsory for sailors to have a daily ration of citrus juice, usually made from lemons or limes. Since them the British have been referred to as 'Limeys'. Lind, in *A Treatise of the Scurvy*, demonstrated the importance of lemon juice. As with most discoveries in medicine or in health, it took the Royal Navy almost *fifty years* to catch on to the importance of such fruits and in 1795 the daily issue of lemon juice was made compulsory.

Sources: all fresh fruits and vegetables; legumes, liver, organ meats.

Vitamin D

Deficiency: Rickets, backache, tooth decay, muscle cramps, dry skin, hair loss.

Discovered by McCollum in 1922, Vitamin D is made in the skin under exposure to sunlight. It can also be found in some foods. As Vitamin A, Vitamin D overdose can be toxic.

Sources: cod liver oil, fish, milk, egg yolks, livers of animals and fish.

Vitamin E

Deficiency: loss of sex drive, oedema, sweating, exhaustion after gentle exercise, easy bruising, infertility, varicose veins, dry skin, puffy ankles, breathing difficulties.

First isolated in 1936 by Evans.

Sources: in most foodstuffs. Best sources: wheatgerm and most oils (always get unrefined, cold-pressed, oils).

Vitamin F

A term no longer in use. Describes essential forms of fats, including linoleic, linolenic and arachidonic acids, and gammalinolenic acid (GLA) and eicosapentaenoic acid (EPA). First described by Burr and Burr in 1929.

Vitamin G

Another extinct term. It is the old-fashioned name for Riboflavin (Vitamin B2).

Vitamin K

Deficiency: lack of blood-clotting mechanism, such as in haemophilia.

First isolated in yellow oil in 1939 by Karrer, Dam, and co-workers.

Sources: spinach, cauliflower, cabbage, meat and milk.

Vitamin P

Another term no longer in common use. They are known better as the bioflavonoids.

First discovered by Gyorgi in 1926.

Source: citrus fruits.

Minerals and Trace Elements

CALCIUM
An essential mineral for strong bone formation and development. Calcium has similar biochemical activities to the vitamins as well as being used for structural components of the body. The human body contains over 3 pounds of calcium; 99 percent of which is in the bones and teeth. The remaining 1 percent is responsible for the strength of the membranes between the cells and also is a co-factor in many enzyme reactions. When Calcium is low, the muscles and nerves become more tense and excitable.

Sources: dairy produce. Nuts, lean meat, chicken, vegetables, whole grains, brewer's yeast.

CHROMIUM
Chromium has been known to play a role in the prevention of cardiovascular disease and is instrumental in regulating blood sugar levels.

Sources: whole grains and cereals. Nuts. Brewer's yeast.

COBALT
Intricately involved with vitamin B12 (cyanacobalamin). Vitamin B12 is the only vitamin to contain a metal – cobalt. A deficiency of either B12 or cobalt can result in pernicious anaemia.

Sources: as Vitamin B12 – animal protein foods.

COPPER
Required for proper pigmentation of skin and hair; the elastic qualities of blood vessels, and the structural integrity of the bones and nerves.

Sources: shellfish, organ meats, nuts, seeds, dairy produce.

IODINE
This essential mineral is needed by the thyroid gland in order to produce the thyroid hormones. A deficiency

produces goiter and many of the same symptoms associated with hypothyroidism: Slow metabolism, mental sluggishness, obesity, dry skin and hair, and other symptoms.

Sources: vegetables, all sea foods.

IRON
Essential mineral responsible for normal haemoglobin formation. A deficiency leads to anaemia.

Sources: red meats, liver, eggs, wheat germ, molasses, plums, cherries, and green leafy vegetables.

MAGNESIUM
Important mineral essential for proper calcium and vitamin C metabolism. It supports healthy levels of nerve and muscle excitability and prevents tremors, spasms, convulsions, and cramps. A deficiency will produce delirium, mental confusion, jerky movements and hypersensitivity to light. An excess of magnesium may produce stupor, low blood pressure and respiratory failure.

Sources: whole grains, nuts, brown rice, fruits, vegetables.

MANGANESE
A mineral necessary for tissue respiration, reproduction, and proper glandular function, especially milk formation in lactating women. Manganese combines with the enzyme phosphatase in bone formation.

Sources: green, leafy vegetables, whole grains, beans, peas, nuts, eggs, and red meats.

MOLYBDENUM
Although rare in the body, it is an essential nutrient, acting as a co-factor in several enzyme systems – particularly energy production.

Sources: beans, peas, wholegrain cereals, leafy vegetables, liver and kidney, fruits and vegetables.

PHOSPHORUS
Phosphorus is present in all of the cells of the body. It is necessary for the utilisation of oxygen by the cells, and is therefore essential to life. Also involved in the metabolism of starches and fats.

Sources: most foods contain phosphorus.

POTASSIUM
Vital to maintain life itself. The human body carries around half a pound of potassium − all of it in the soft tissues or fluids of the body. A severe deficiency manifests itself in muscular weakness, paralysis, difficult breathing, and cardiac irregularities. Any excess is automatically excreted in the urine.

Sources: most foods contain potassium.

SELENIUM
Important antioxidant and immune system stimulant. Many bodily functions depend on this trace mineral, including the muscles, hair, skin, nails, and red blood cells. It is also involved in the production of sperm.

Sources: wholegrain cereals, nuts, vegetables, fruits, milk, meats.

SILICON
The most abundant mineral on earth. Parts of the body particularly dependent on an adequate supply are the brain, heart, muscles, hair, ligaments, liver, lungs, bones and blood vessels. Easily excreted in the urine.

Sources: most foods contain silicon.

ZINC
Without zinc, the cells could not breathe, grow, or reproduce. This essential mineral plays a very important role in male sexual potency. Zinc supplements have also been shown to be helpful in treating acne and rheumatoid arthritis.

Sources: whole grains, all fish, liver, beef, peas, corn, eggs, carrots, milk, rice.

DEFICIENCY STATES
Table 3. Signs known to be of value in nutrition surveys and their interpretation (Kanawati, A.A. (1976) from *Nutrition in the Community*, ed. McLaren, D.S., John Wiley & Sons Ltd: Chichester.)

Signs	Associated disorder of Nutrient
Hair	
Lack of lustre	Protein energy malnutrition
Thinness and sparseness*	Protein energy malnutrition
Straightness	Protein energy malnutrition
Dyspigmentation*	Protein energy malnutrition
(Abnormal hair colouring)	
Flag sign	Protein energy malnutrition
(Abnormal colour in patches)	
Easy Pluckability*	Protein energy malnutrition
Face	
Naso-labial dyssebacea	Riboflavin
(Dysfunction of upper lip sweat gland; usually sweating)	
Moon-face	Kwashiorkor
Eyes	
Dry Eyes*	Vitamin A
Conjunctival xerosis*	Vitamin A
(Abnormal dryness of eye lining: Bitot's spots)	
Corneal xerosis	Vitamin A
(Abnormal dryness of cornea)	
Keratomalacia*	Vitamin A
(Thickening of eye tissue)	
Lips	
Angular stomatitis*	Riboflavin
(Cracks at corner of mouth)	
Angular scars	Riboflavin
(Scarring at corner of mouth)	
Cheilosis*	Riboflavin
(Maceration at corners of mouth)	
Tongue	
Scarlet and raw tongue*	Nicotinic acid
Magenta tongue	Riboflavin
Teeth	
Mottled enamel*	Fluorosis
Gums	
Spongy bleeding gums*	Ascorbic acid

Table 3 continued

Glands
Thyroid enlargement*   Iodine
Parotid enlargement   Starvation
(Enlargement of mumps gland)

Skin
Xerosis   Vitamin A
(Abnormal dryness)
Perifollicular Hyperkeratosis*   Vitamin A
(Crusts at base of hair follicles)
Petechiae   Ascorbic acid
(Small capilliary bleeding)
Pellagrous dermatosis*   Nicotinic Acid
(Inflammation with eruptions)
Flaky paint dermatosis*   Kwashiorkor
(Inflammation with flaking)
Scrotal and vulval dermatosis   Riboflavin
(Inflammation of skin at genital areas)

Nails
Koilonychia   Iron
(Thickening and ridging)

Subcutaneous tissue
Oedema*   Kwashiorkor
(Fluid retention)
Fat decreased   Starvation, marasmus
Fat increased   Obesity

Muscular and skeletal systems
Muscle wasting*   Starvation, marasmus,
                                                        kwashiorkor
Craniotabes   Vitamin D
(Mis-shaping of skull in development)
Frontal and parietal bossing   Vitamin D
(Bowing out at front and/or side of head)
Epiphyseal enlargement*   Vitamin D
(Increase in size of growing ends of bone)
Beading of ribs   Vitamin D
Persistently open anterior fontanelle*   Vitamin D
(Incomplete skull development)
Knock-knees or bow legs*   Vitamin D
Thoracic rosary   Vitamin D, ascorbic acid
(Rash surrounding chest)
Musculo-skeletal haemorrhages   Ascorbic Acid
(Bleeding into muscle tissues and joints)

Internal systems
(a) Gastro intestinal
Hepatomegaly*   Kwashiorkor
(Enlarged liver)

(b) Nervous
Psychomotor changes   Kwashiorkor
(Incoordinated muscle activity associated with
mental disturbance)
Mental confusion   Thiamine, nicotinic acid
Sensory loss   Thiamine, nicotinic acid
Motor weakness   Thiamine, nicotinic acid
(Reduced power of limbs)

Table 3 continued

Loss of position sense	Thiamine, nicotinic acid
Loss of vibration	Thiamine
Loss of ankle and knee jerks	Thiamine
Calf tenderness	Thiamine
Cardiac	
Cardiac enlargement	Thiamine
Tachycardia	Thiamine
(Abnormally rapid heart)	

*Suggested for use in a rapid survey.

There are more serious and life-threatening deficiencies which we often see on our T.V. screens in the likes of Ethiopia or Sudan. These are deficiency *syndromes*, which I describe below:

Marasmus and Kwashiorkor

These are deficiency conditions referred to as PEM (Protein Energy Malnutrition). This is a widespread spectrum of disease with its severe forms manifesting themselves as Marasmus and Kwashiorkor. There is no precise way of defining subclinical forms that can be characterised by retardation of growth and development. A large proportion of the several hundred million pre-school children in the developing world are affected to some degree. There is a deficiency of energy and all nutrients in marasmus, while kwashiorkor results from deficiency of protein and to a lesser extent other nutrients in the presence of adequate or even excess energy intake. Marasmus is really starvation in the child.

General features	Marasmus	Kwashiorkor
Occurrence:	World-wide	Limited
Usual Age:	Infancy	2nd and 3rd years
Adaptation to stress:	Good	Poor
Response to treatment		
immediate:	Poor	Good (Occasional sudden death)
ultimate:	Fair	Good
Long-Term effects		
mental:	Severe	Less severe

physical:	Severe	Mild
liver damage:	Nil	Nil
Clinical signs		
Oedema:	Absent	Present
Dermatosis:	Rare	Common
Hair Changes:	Common	Very Common
Hepatomegaly:	Common	Very Common
Mental changes:	Uncommon	Very Common
Wasting of fat/muscles:	Severe	Mild
Stunting:	Severe	Moderate
Anaemia:	Common/severe	Mild
Vitamin deficiencies:	Uncommon	Common

In July 1991, the British government's new report 'Dietary Reference Values for Food Energy and Nutrients for the United Kingdom' was published. It effectively abolished the Recommended Daily Amounts (RDA) which had been used as a measure of dietary standards since World War II. The term RDA has been replaced by the Dietary Reference Value (DRV) – a blanket term which in fact refers to *three* new sets of figures. Each of these sets of figures in turn has its own name. These are as follows:

Reference Nutrient Intake (RNI): This is roughly equivalent to (but in most cases lower than) the old RDA. The RNI figures for the various nutrients are assumed to meet the needs of all healthy people except for a very small percentage with exceptionally high requirements.

The Estimated Average Requirement (EAR): The EAR figures for the various nutrients are assumed to meet the requirements of all healthy people with average nutritional needs.

The Lower Reference Nutrient Intake (LRNI): According to the report, 'Intakes below this level are almost certainly inadequate for most individuals'.

Dietary Reference Values for Vitamins and Minerals

Dietary Reference Values for Vitamins and Minerals

	Old RDA*	RNI*	EAR*	LRNI*
		given as daily amounts		
Vitamins				
Vitamin A	750ug	700ug	500ug	300ug
Thiamine (B1)	1.2mg**	1.0mg	0.3mg	0.23mg
Riboflavin (B2)	1.6mg	1.3mg	1.0mg	0.8mg
Niacin (B3)	18mg	17mg	5.5mg	4.4mg
Pyridoxine (B6)	–	1.4mg++	1.2mg++	1.0mg++
Cyanocobalamin (B12)	–	1.5ug	1.25ug	1.0ug
Folic Acid	–	200ug	150ug	100ug
Vitamin C	30mg	40mg	25mg	10mg
Minerals				
Calcium	500mg	750mg	525mg	400mg
Phosphorus	–	550mg	400mg	310mg
Magnesium	–	300mg	250mg	190mg
Sodium	–	1600mg	–	575mg
Potassium	–	3500mg	–	2000mg
Chloride	–	2500mg	–	885mg
Iron	10mg	8.7mg	6.7mg	4.7mg
Zinc	–	9.5mg	7.3mg	5.5mg
Copper	–	1.2mg	–	–
Selenium	–	75ug	–	40ug
Iodine	–	140ug	–	70ug

DRV's for protein, fat, sugars and starches, energy (calories), and non-starch polysaccharides (dietary fibre) have also been devised, and can be found in summary form in Dietary Reference Values – a Guide.

* These are the figures for males aged 19–50 years.
** This is the figure for moderately active young men.
++ Based on a daily protein intake of 14.7% of total energy (calories).

Table by kind permission of Linda Lazarides, Secretary of the SPNT (The Society for the Promotion of Nutritional Therapy).

Useful Addresses

(U.K., U.S.A., Germany, Spain, Mexico, Argentina)

U.K.

The McCarrison Society

For details, please contact:

Professor M. Crawford
Institute of Brain Chemistry and Nutrition
Queen Elizabeth Hospital for Children
Hackney Road
London E2 8PS

Disseminates and promotes the work of Sir Robert McCarrison, most famous for his study on the health of the Hunzas.

The Gerson Therapy in Great Britain

For details, contact:

Mrs Pat Faulkner
The Flat, Woodbrook House
Killanne
Enniscorthy
Co. Wexford, Ireland

Tel: 00-353-5455114

Pat Faulkner is the British contact for anyone interested in the Gerson Therapy; a wonderful nutritional approach to all health disorders, including cancer.

Action Against Allergy
24/26 High Street
Hampton Hill
Middlesex TW12 1PD

AAA is the leading organisation disseminating information on all aspects of food/chemical/inhalant allergies.
It is a charity and you should ensure an S.A.E. is enclosed
if you wish a reply. They have a large stock of books on
food allergies and nutrition.

The York Nutritional Laboratory
Dept. ABAP
Tudor House
Lysander Close
Clifton Moore
York

Tel: 01990-100812

Long established nutritional laboratory who perform
blood tests for food allergies as well as other nutritionally-
oriented services.

Society for the Promotion of Nutritional Therapy (SPNT)
1st Floor,
The Enterprise Centre,
Station Parade,
Eastbourne BN21 1BE

Tel: 01323 430203

Holds a register of nutritional therapists and will advise
on seeking courses on nutrition. You may contact them
for a register of their members.

Nutrition Consultants' Association
20 Alexandra Ave
Southall,
Middx. UB1 2AL

Tel: 0181 574-7098

Holds a register of consultants and may be contacted for same.

The British College of Nutritional Medicine
East Bank
New Church Road
Smithills
Greater Manchester
BL1 5QP

Tel: 01884-255059

Holds recognised diploma courses for qualification in Nutritional Medicine and can supply register of their graduates.

Institute for Optimum Nutrition
5 Jerdan Place
London SW6 1BE

Tel: 0181-877-9993

Holds recognised diploma courses for qualification as a Nutrition Consultant and can supply register of their graduates.

General Council and Register of Naturopaths
6 Netherhall Gardens
London NW3 5RR

Tel: 0171-435-8728

Holds recognised full-time courses for qualification in Naturopathy, which includes excellent dietary training.

British Complementary Medical Association
St. Charles Hospital
Exmoor Street
London W10 6DZ

Tel: 0171-964-1205

Holds register of practitioners in various complementary disciplines and you can telephone for this information.

The Nutri Centre
Hale Clinic
7 Park Crescent
London W1N 3HE

Tel: 0171-436-5122

The Hale Clinic houses the Nutri Centre downstairs which claims not only to have the largest and most up-to-date selection of British and American food allergy and nutritionally-oriented books in the U.K. but make an identical claim for their massive range of nutritional supplements.

Wholefoods
24 Paddington Street
London W1M 4DR

Tel: 0171-935-3924

An excellent wholefood shop which sells not only organic produce but many books on allergies, diet and nutrition, as well as nutritional supplements.

Hanover Health Foods
40 Hanover Street
Edinburgh EH2 2DR

Tel: 0131-225-4291

A good nutritional supplements shop should you ever go to Edinburgh.

Here's Health
Victory House
14 Leicester Place
London WC2H 7BP

Tel: 0171-437-9011

Monthly magazine devoted to healthy living with emphasis placed on 'alternative' therapies and success stories. Also contains lists of associations and practitioners of most disciplines.

Journal of Alternative and Complementary Medicine
Green Library
Homewood House
Guildford Road
Chertsey
Surrey KT16 0QA

Tel: 01932-874333

To quote from their publication: 'The only independent monthly in the world devoted to unorthodox therapy and treatments.' They have many medical doctors on their editorial board of advisers.

Hyperactive Children's Support Group
71 Whyke Lane
Chichester
W. Sussex
PO19 2LD

Tel: 01903-725182

They offer advice to parents with hyperactive children; often advising them to look at their children's diets for possible food or chemical allergies as being causative.

Slimming Magazine
EMAP Elan
Victory House
Leicester Place
London WC2H 7BP

Tel 0171-437-9011

Self explanatory: Devoted to issues on slimming.

The Hale Clinic
7 Park Crescent
London W1N 3HE

Tel: 0171-631-0156

A multi-discipline clinic in central London.

Bio-Health Ltd
Culpepper Close
Medway City Estate
Rochester, Kent ME2 4HU

Tel: 01634-290115

Large range of nutritional supplements and services.

Lamberts Healthcare Ltd
1 Lamberts Road
Tunbridge Wells
Kent
TN2 3EQ

Tel: 01892-513116
Large range of nutritional supplements and services
available.

Cantassium Ltd
225 Putney Bridge Road
London SW15 2PY

Tel: 0181-874-1130

Wide range of nutritional supplements available.

Rosemary Cartwright Dip ION
London Road
Forest Row
East Sussex RH18 5EZ

Tel: 01342-82-2716

Graduate of the Institute of Optimum Nutrition and has
good range of products on her premises.

Mike Franklin (Author of book on M.E.)
The Oxford Nutritional Therapy Practice
28 Aysgarth Road
Yarnton

Oxford
OX5 1ND

Tel: 01865-375923

T.H. Jivraj B.Sc.
286 Preston Road
Harrow, Middx HA3 0BZ

Tel: 0181-908-4272

Practises homeopathy and nutrition.

A.G. Dickenson M.BR.Ac.A.
Chester Allergy Clinic
Warwick House
4 Stanley Place
Chester CH1 2LU

Tel: 01244-318963

Acupuncture and allergy practitioner.

Wholistic Research Company
Bright Haven
Robin's Lane
Lolworth
Cambridge
CB3 8HH

Tel: 01954-781074

Suppliers of 'Champion' and 'Norwalk' juicers as well
as a large selection of books and other equipment for
'alternative' therapies.

Organic Farm Foods (Scotland) Ltd
Block 7
Whiteside Industrial Estate
Bathgate
West Lothian
EH48 2RX

Tel: 01506-632750

Suppliers of organic fruits and vegetables.

USEFUL ADDRESSES: U.S.A.

The Gerson Institute
P.O. Box 430
Bonita, California USA

Tel (619)-472-7450

The Gerson Therapy Clinic's American offices.

The American Holistic Medical Association
4101 Lake Boone Trail
Suite 201
Raleigh
North Carolina 27607

Tel: (919) 787-5146

They supply names of doctors who are naturopathically-oriented.

The World Research Foundation
15300 Ventura Blvd
Suite 405
Sherman Oaks, California 91403

Tel: (818)-907-5483

They have a list of 255 organisations, health professionals, hospitals and clinics worldwide as well as a huge database covering 5,000 medical journals on health problems and the options open for treatment.

The American Association of Naturopathic Physicians has a free referral service.
Phone them on Tel: (206)-323-7610.

Price-Pottenger Nutrition Foundation
PO Box 2614
La Mesa
California 92044-0702

Tel: (619)-582-4168

They disseminate and promote all aspects of nutrition and health, in particular the findings of Weston A. Price D.D.S. who published his famous work 'Nutrition and Physical Degeneration' – available from the foundation.

The Princeton Brain Bio Center
862 Route 518
Skillman
Njer 08558

Tel: (609)-924-8607

This is a food allergy clinic.

Boston Orthomolecular Society Inc
c/o 132 Topsfield Road
Boxford, MA 01921

Tel: (617) 887-5062

An organization concerned with the orthomolecular (megadoses of nutrients) approach in the treatment of many disorders.

The Huxley Institute for Biosocial Research
900 North Federal Highway
Boca Raton, FL 33432

Tel: (800)-847-3802

Concerned with nutrition health and human behaviour. Serves as a referral service for information on orthomolecular physicians and health practitioners in the USA and holds annual medical symposia and training sessions for the education of physicians and laypersons in the field of nutrition and health.

Bay'n Gulf Hygienic Home
18207-09 Gulf Boulevard
Redington Shores
St. Petersburg, Florida 33708

USA

Fasting clinic.

Esser's Hygienic Rest Ranch
PO Box 161
Lake Worth
Florida 33460
USA

Fasting Clinic

Shelton's Health School
PO Box 1277
San Antonio
Texas 78295
USA

Probably the longest established fasting clinic in America.

Ehret Literature Publishing Company Inc
19 Babcock Place
Yonkers, NY 10701
USA

Books and information on the works of Professor Arnold Ehret.

Norwalk Press
107 North Cortez
Suite 200
Prescott, AZ 86301
USA

Books and information on the works of Dr. Norman W. Walker who advocated raw vegetable juices and died recently at 110!

Health Science
Box 7
Santa Barabara, Calif 93102
USA

Books on diet, health and fasting by Paul and Patricia Bragg, naturopaths.

Feingold Association of the US
PO Box 6550
Alexandria VA 22306

International College of Applied Nutrition
Referral Service
312 E. Las Tunas Drive
San Gabriel, Calif, 91776
USA

Pawling Health Manor
PO Box 401
Hyde Park, N.Y. 12538
USA

Fasting Clinic

MEXICO

CHIPSA
449 Nubes
Playas de Tijuana
Mexico

Tel: 011-516-680-2910

Gerson hospital facility in Mexico.

Villa Vegetariana
PO Box 1228
Cuernavaca
Mexico

Fasting Clinic

ARGENTINA

The Cormillot Clinic
Paraguay 3358

Buenos Aires
Argentina

Fasting Clinic

GERMANY

Clinic Dr. Otto Buchinger
Clinic for Biological Therapy
Nutrition and Metabolic Diseases
D-3280 Bad Pyrmont – Forstweg 39

Tel: (0 52 81) 16 60

Fasting Clinic

Buchinger-Klinik am Bodensee
777 Uberlingen
Lake Constance
Germany

Fasting Clinic

AUSTRALIA

SOMA is a health association located in Australia. They produce detailed monthly newsletters emphasising research in nutrition and biochemistry in physical and mental illness.

SOMA Health Association of Australia Ltd
GPO Box 3745
Sydney, NSW 2001
Australia

SPAIN

Clinica Buchinger
Marbella, SA
Marbella (Malaga)
Spain

Fasting Clinic

Suggested Reading

Books on Food Allergies and/or Nutrition

The Colon Health Handbook, Robert Gray: Emerald Pub, Nevada

The Complete Raw Juice Therapy, Susan E. Charmine: Thorsons, London

Cures That Work, Janet Pleshette: Century Arrow, London

Natural Therapeutics, Vols I II III. Henry Lindlahr: The C.W. Daniel Co., Saffron Walden

Fasting for Renewal of Life, Herbert M. Shelton: Natural Hygiene Press, Chicago

The Pulse Test, Arthur F. Coca M.D.: Arco Publishing, New York

Not All In The Mind, Richard Mackarness: Pan Books, London

Chemical Victims, Richard Mackarness: Pan Books, London

Brain Allergies, Wm. Philpott and D. Kalita: Keats Pub, USA

Nutrition and Physical Degeneration, Weston A. Price: Keats Publishing, USA

Food in Antiquity, Don and Patricia Brothwell: Thames and Hudson, London

A Cancer Therapy (Results of Fifty Cases), Max Gerson M.D. Gerson Institute, Bonita, Calif, USA

Enzyme Nutrition, Dr. Edward Howell. Avery Pubshg, New Jersey, USA

Unconventional Medicine, New English Library, U.K.

Nutritional Influences on Mental Illness, Melvyn R. Werbach M.D. Third Line Press, Tarzana, Calif, USA

Nutritional Influences on Illness, Melvyn Werbach: Third Line Press, Tanzana, Calif, USA

Hunza Health Secrets, Renee Taylor: Keats Pub, USA

Fasting: The Ultimate Diet. Alan Cott M.D.: Bantam Books, New York

How to Live Longer and Feel Better, Linus Pauling. W.H. Freeman and Co, New York

Encyclopaedia of Alternative Medicine and Self-Help, Malcolm Hulke. Rider & Co, London.

Naturopathic Medicine, Roger Newman Turner. Thorsons. U.K.

Fasting: The Buchinger Method, M. Wilhemi-Buchinger: The C.W. Daniel Co. Saffron Walden.

Life Food Juices, H.E. Kirschner M.D.: H.E. Kirschner Publications, Monrovia, Calif. USA.

Dr. Atkin's Diet Revolution. Robert C. Atkins M.D. Bantam Press. New York.

The Stone-Age Health Programme, Eaton, Shostak, and Konner: Angus and Robertson. NSW. Australia.

10 Day Clean-Up Plan, Leslie Kenton. Century, London.

Fasting, Shirley Ross. Sheldon Press. London.

Fasting Can Save Your Life. Shelton. ANHS Publications. Tampa, Florida, USA.

Instinctive Nutrition, Schaeffer: Celestial Arts, Calif. USA.

Dr. Atkins' Nutrition Breakthrough, Robert C. Atkins M.D. Bantam Books, New York.

The Miracle of Fasting, Paul C. Bragg: Health Science. Santa Barbara, Calif. USA.

Candida Albicans, Leon Chaitow. Thorsons. U.K.

Solved: The Riddle of Illness, Langer and Scheer: Keats Pubshg. Conn. USA.

The Migraine Revolution, Dr. John Mansfield. Thorsons, U.K.

How To Control Your Allergies, Robert Forman Ph.D: Larchmont Books. New York.

Cancer Winner, Jaquie Davison: Midwest Press, Mo. USA.

How to Fortify Your Immune System, Donald Dickenson: Arlington Books, London.

Food Allergy, Rita Greer and Robert Woodward. Roberts Publctns. London.

Feasting on Raw Foods, Ed: Charles Gerras: Thorsons, U.K.

About Fasting, Otto H.F. Buchinger M.D.: Thorsons, U.K.

Food Facts and Fallacies. Fredericks and Bailey. Arco. New York.

Nutrition and Mental Illness. Carl C. Pfeiffer M.D.: Healing Arts Press, Vt. USA.

The Food Allergy Plan. Keith Mumby: Unwin. London.

Overfed but Undernourished, Dr. Curtis Wood Jr: Tower Publications. New York.

Super Natural Immune Power. Weller: Thorsons. U.K.

The Healthy Human Gut, C. Leslie Thomson: Thomson-Kingston Publications, Edinburgh.

The Manual of Natural Living, Barreau and Salomon: Thorsons.

New Hope for Incurable Diseases. Cheraskin and Ringsdorf: Arco. New York.

Nerve Troubles, Science of Life Books. Melbourne, Australia.

Cancer? Think Curable: The Gerson Therapy. Gerson Institute. Bonita, California.

A Guide to the Nervous System, John Gibson: Faber and Faber, London.

Dr. Schuessler's Biochemistry, J.B. Chapman M.D. Thorsons. UK.

Against the Unsuspected Enemy, Amelia Nathan Hill, New Horizon. Bognor Regis.

The Complete Home Guide to all the Vitamins, Ruth Adams: Larchmont Books. New York.

The Allergy Handbook, Dr. Keith Mumby. Thorsons. U.K.

Let's Eat Right to Keep Fit, Adelle Davis: Unwin Books. New York.

I Fought Leukemia – and Won!, Rex B. Eyre: Hawkes Publishing Salt Lake City. USA.

The Bircher-Benner Health Guide, Ruth Kunz-Bircher: Unwin Paperbacks. London.

Goodbye to Arthritis, Patricia Byrivers: Century Arrow. London

DLPA The Natural Pain Killer and Anti-Depressant, Dr. Arnold Fox and Barry Fox: Thorsons U.K.

The Complete Scarsdale Medical Diet, Herman Tarnower M.D. & Samm Baker. Bantam. New York.

Your Daily Diet, Capt. Geoffrey T. Whitehouse. Here's Health Guide Books: Newman Turner Publications. U.K.

Let's Stay Healthy, Adelle Davis. Unwin. New York.

The food Intolerance Diet Book, Workman, Jones, Hunter: Martin Dunitz. London.

Food for Fitness, World Publications. Mt. View. Calif. USA.

Homeopathy and Your Emotions, Sheila Harrison: Ashgrove Press. Bath, U.K.

The Allergy Connection. Barbara Paterson: Thorsons. U.K.

Megavitamin Therapy. Ruth Adams and Frank Murray: Larchmont Books. New York.

Diet and Salad, Dr. Norman W. Walker, D.Sc: Norwalk Press, USA.

Raw Energy. Leslie and Susannah Kenton. Arrow Books. London.

How to Improve Your Digestion and Absorption. Christopher Scarfe: ION Press. London.

The Bristol Diet, Dr. Alec Forbes. Century Arrow. London.

How to Get Rid of the Poisons in your Body: Gary and Steven Null: Arco. New York.

Skin Troubles, Leon Chaitow N.D.: Thorsons. U.K.

Let's Cook it Right, Adelle Davis. Unwin Paperbacks. New York.

How to Live With Hypoglycemia, Charles Weller M.D.: Jove Publtns, New York.

A Natural Approach; Allergies, Michio Kushi: Japan Publications. New York.

Improve Your Sight Without Glasses, Science of Life Books. Melbourne. Australia.

The Allergy Problem, Vicky Rippere M.A.: Thorsons. U.K.

Let's Get Well, Adelle Davis: Unwin. New York.

Mucusless Diet Healing System, Prof. Arnold Ehret: Ehret Lit. Publishing. Yonkers, NY.

The Food Depression Connection, June Roth: Contemporary Books. Chicago. USA.

Nutrition and the Mind, George Watson M.D.: California. USA.

Dr. Atkins' Super Energy Diet, Robert C. Atkins: Bantam New York.

A Time to Heal. Beata Bishop: Hodder and Stoughton. U.K.

The Cambridge Diet, Alan Howard: Corgi Books. London.

The Healing Crisis. C. Leslie Thomson: Thomson-Kingston Publications, Edinburgh.

In Search of The Perfect Cleanse. Jason Winters: Vinton Pub. Las Vegas. Nev. USA.

Low Blood Sugar. Martin L. Budd N.D.: Thorsons U.K.

Eat Fat and Grow Slim. Richard Mackarness. Fontana. London.

Body, Mind and the B Vitamins. Ruth Adams and Frank Murray. Larchmont Books. New York.

This Slimming Business. John Yudkin: Penguin Books. London.

Allergic to Food? Rita Greer: J.M. Dent & Sons. London.

Nutrition and Disease, Ed: R.J. Jarrett: Croom Helm. London.

Vibrant Health. Dr. N.W. Walker: Norwalk Press. Arizona. USA.

A Doctor's Proven New Home Cure for Arthritis, Giraud Campbell Thorsons, U.K.

Success Against Allergy, Mary Simpson: Simpson Graphics. Balerno, Edinburgh.

Evening Primrose Oil, Judy Graham: Thorsons, U.K.

Magnesium, the Nutrient That Could Change Your Life: J. Rodale Pyramid Books. New York.

Improve Your Health with Zinc, Ruth Adams and Frank Murray: Larchmont Books. New York.

Overcoming Addictions. Janette Pleshette: Thorsons. U.K.

Rational Fasting, Prof. Arnold Ehret. Ehret Publishing, Yonkers New York.

Nutrition and Its Disorders, Donald S. McLaren: Churchill Livingstone, Edinburgh.

The Secrets of Successful Fasting, Dr. H. Lutzner: Thorsons, UK.

A Matter of Life, Dr. N. Coates and N. Jollyman: MacDonald & Co. London.

Food Allergy and Intolerance, Dr. J. Brostoff and L. Gamlin: Bloomsbury Publishing. London.

Nutrition and Health, The McCarrison Society. London.

The Amino Revolution. Dr. R. Erdmann and M. Jones: Century. London.

Ultra Health, Leslie Kenton: Arrow Books. London.

The Super Supplements Bible, Dr. Rosenbaum and D. Bosco: Thorsons, U.K.

Mental Illness and Schizophrenia, Dr. Carl Pfeiffer: Thorsons, U.K.

Colon Health, Dr Norman W. Walker: Norwalk Press. Ariz. USA.

Become Younger, Dr. Norman W. Walker: Norwalk Press. Ariz. USA.

The Shocking Truth About Water. Patricia and Paul C. Bragg: Health Science. Calif. USA.

The Grape Cure. Joanna Brandt: Ehret Literature Co. Yonkers. New York.

Daniel: Living With an Allergic Child, Diana Wells. Ashgrove Press, Bath. U.K.

Clinical Ecology, Dr. G. Lewith and Dr. J. Kenyon: Thorsons UK.

Pottenger's Cats, Francis M. Pottenger Jr. M.D.: Price-Pottenger Nutrition Foundation. Calif. USA.

Psycho-Nutrition, Carlton Fredericks Ph.D: Putnam Publishing. New York.

Vitamin Vitality, Patrick Holford: Collins, London.

Clear Body Clear Mind, Leon Chaitow: Unwin Paperbacks. London.

Minerals: Kill or Cure? Adams and Murray: Larchmont. New York.

Body, Mind, and Sugar. E.M. Abrahamson and A.W. Pezet: Avon Books. New York.

Goodbye Allergies, Judge Tom Blaine. Zebra Books. New York.

Dr. Mandell's Five-Day Allergy Relief System, M. Mandell and L.W. Scanlon: Crowell. New York.

Food Allergy: Provocative Testing and Injection Therapy, J.B. Miller: Charles C. Thomas. Springfield. Ill. USA.

Fighting Depression, Harvey M. Ross M.D.: Larchmont. New York.

Raw Vegetable Juices. Dr. Norman Walker: Jove Books. New York.

The Grape Cure, Basil Shackleton. Thorsons Publishers. U.K.

Philosophy of Natural Therapeutics, Henry Lindlahr M.D.: The C.W. Daniel Co. Ltd. Saffron Walden. U.K.

Tracking Down Hidden Food Allergies, W.G. Crook: Professional Books. Tenn. USA.

References

1. Davis, Adelle. Let's Stay Healthy. Unwin Paperbacks. London 1983.
2. Langer, Stephen E. and Scheer, James F: Solved: The Riddle of Illness. Keats Publishing. Conn. U.S.A. 1984.
3. Budd, Martin L.: Low Blood Sugar. Thorsons. 1984.
4. Coca, Arthur F.: The Pulse Test, ARC Books. New York. 1972.
5. Mansfield, John: The Migraine Revolution. Thorsons 1987.
6. Adams, Ruth and Murray, Frank: Minerals: Kill or Cure? Larchmont books, New York 1974.
7. Greer, Rita and Woodward, Robert: Food Allergy – A Practical Easy Guide: Roberts Publications, London 1982.
8. Byrivers, Patricia: Goodbye to Arthritis: Century Arrow, London 1987.
9. Sansum, W.D.: The Treatment of Indigestion, Underweight and Allergy with the Old and New forms of Digestive Agents, 1932.
10. Howell, Edward: Enzyme Nutrition: Avery Publishing, Njer 1985.
11. Lewith, George T. et al., Clinical Ecology. Thorsons 1985.
12. Donsbach, Kurt W.: Allergies: Int. Inst. of Nat. Health Sciences, Calif. U.S.A. 1977.
13. Weller, Stella: Super Natural Immune Power: Thorsons 1989.
14. Davis, Adelle: Let's Get Well: Unwin Books, London 1985.
15. Jarrett, R.J. Nutrition and Disease. Croom Helm Ltd, London 1979.
16. Bullen, C.L. et al: J. Med. Microbiol. (1977) 10; 403–13.
17. Pauling, Linus: How to Live Longer and Feel Better: W.H. Freeman & Co. New York. 1986.
18. Atkins, Robert C.: Nutrition Breakthrough. Bantam, New York. 1981.

19. Chandra, R.K. Immunodeficiency in undernutrition and over-nutrition. Nutrition Reviews. June 1982: 39(6): 255–31.

20. Suskind, R.M.: Malnutrition and the Immune Response: Raven Press. 1977.

21. Chandra, R.K., Joshi, P., et al: Nutrition and immunocompetence of the elderly. Effect of short term nutritional supplementation on cell-mediated immunity and lymphocyte subsets: Nutrition Research, 1982: 2: 223–32.

22. Ludovici, P.P. et al; Proc. Soc. Exp. Biol. Med: 77, 526; 1951.

23. Axelrod, A.E., Nut. Rev. 10,353;1952.

24. Axelrod, A.E., et al., Ann. New York. Aca. Sci; 63,202: 1955.

25. Kenton, Leslie and Susannah: Raw Energy. Century Arrow, 1986.

26. Ward, Brian: The Body and Health: MacDonald Educational Ltd. 1978.

27. Thomson, James, C.: The Healthy Human Gut: Kingston Publtns 1986.

28. Howard, Edward: Enzyme Nutrition: Avery Pub. Njer. 1985.

29. Jochems, Ruth: The Dr. Moerman Cancer Diet: Sheldon Press, London 1989.

30. Anthony, Michael: Research in Clinical Studies in Headache (1978) Vol. 6: pp110–16.

31. Blundell, J.E.: Serotonin and Appetite: Neuropharmacology 1984: 23: 1536–51.

32. Cangiano, C., Cascino, A. et al. Plasma and CSF tryptophan in cancer anorexia. J. Neural. Transm: 1990; 81: 225–33.

33. Rossi-Fanelli, F.: Cangiano, C.: Increased availability of tryptophan in brain as common pathogenic mechanism for anorexia associated with different diseases: Nutrition, 1991; 7: 364–7.

34. Kirschner, H.E.: Live Food Juices: H.E. Kirschner Pubtns, Calif. 1957.

35. Rosenbaum, Dr. Michael E. and Bosco, Dominick: The Super Supplements Bible: Thorsons. 1987.

36. Int. Jnl. of Obesity (1991): 15: 781–90.

37. Nutrition and Its Disorders: Donald S. McLaren: Churchill Livingstone 1976.

38. Burwell, C.S. et al. Extreme Obesity Associated with Alveolar Hypoventilation – Pickwickian Syndrome. Amer. Jnl. Med. 21: 81–88.

39. Int. Jnl. of Obesity (1986) Vol. 10. No. 5: 349–54.
40. Zelman, S. Arch. Nut. Med. 90, 141. 1952.
41. Westwater, J.O. et al. Gastroenterology 34, 686. 1958.
42. Leevy, C.M. et al. Arch. Int. Med. 92, 527. 1953.
43. Dewey, Kathryn, G: Heinig, M. Jane, et al: Amer. Jnl. of Clin. Nutrition. Feb 1993 Vol 57, No. 2.
44. Shorvan, H.J. and Richardson, J.S. (1949): Sudden obesity and psychological trauma. Br. Med. J: 29, 951–956.
45. Baird, J.B.: Diabetes mellitus and obesity. Proc. Nutr. Soc: 32, 199: (1973).
46. Camstock, G.W., Kendrick, M.A. and Livesay, V.T.: Subcutaneous fatness and mortality. Am. J. Epidemiol: 83, 548 (1966).
47. Gordon, T. and Kannel, W.B: The effects of overweight on cardiovascular disease: Geriatrics: 28, 80 (1973).
48. Marks, H.H.: Influence of obesity on morbidity and mortality. Bull. N.Y. Acadm. Med. 36, 396 (1960).
49. Pooling Project Research Group: Relationship of blood pressure, serum cholesterol, smoking habit, relative weight and ECG abnormalities to incidence of major coronary events: Final report of the Pooling Project. J. CHRON. Dis/ 31, 201 (1978).
50. Stamler, R., Stamler, J., Reidlinger, W., Algera, G. and Roberts, R: Weight and blood pressure. Findings in hypertension screening of one million Americans. J. Am. Med. Asn. 240, 1607 (1978).
51. Peckham, S.C. et al. J. Nut. 77; 187, 1962.
52. Nutrition and its Disorders. 2nd Ed. Donald S. McLaren. Churchill Livingston. 1976.
53. Int. Jnl. of Obesity (1986) 10, 519–525. Physical activity and fitness in obese children. Huttunen, Knip and Paavilainen.
54. Borjeson, M. (1962) Overweight children. Acta. Paediatri. Scand. (Suppl.) 132.
55. Drenick, Ernst, J. (1980); Risk of obesity and surgical indications. Int. Journl. of Obesity: 5, 387–398.
56. Bjorvell, H., Hadell, K., Jonsson, B., Molin, C. and Rossner, S.: Long-term effects of jaw fixation in severe obesity. Int. Jrnl of Obesity. (1984): 8, 79–86.
57. Amer. Jnl. Clin. Nutrition. Supp to Vol 56. No. 1. July 1992: pp 240S–243S.
58. Duncan, G.L., Jenson, W.K. Fraser, R.I. and Cristofori, R.L.: Intermittent fasts in the correction and control of intractable obesity. J. Am. Med. Assn. 181, 309–312: 1962.

59. Cahill, G.F. Jr., Starvation in man, New England J. Med. 282, 668–675; 1970.
60. Bloom, W.L. Fasting as an introduction to the treatment of obesity. Metabolism. 8, 214–220; 1959.
61. Folin, O., Denis, W.: On starvation and obesity with special reference to acidosis. J. Biol. Chem. 21, 183–189: 1915.
62. Wilhelmi-Buchinger; Fasting: The Buchinger Method: C.W. Daniel Co. Ltd. England. 1984.
63. Fredericks, Carlton. Psycho-Nutrition: Pedigree Books: New York. 1976.
64. Kenton, Leslie: Raw Energy; Century Arrow, London 1984.
65. Pottenger, Francis: Pottengers Cats: A Study in Nutrition Price-Pottenger Nutrition Foundation. 1983.
66. Bishop, Beata: A Time to Heal: New English Library 1989.
67. Food for Fitness: World Publications, Calif. 1975.
68. Garber, C.M.: Eating with the Eskimos: Hygeia 16; 242; 1938.
69. Atkins, Robert C., Nutrition Breakthrough. Bantam Books. New York. 1981.
70. Reiser, Raymond: Amer. Jnl. Clin. Nutn: Vol 31. May 1978; 865–75.
71. MacDonald, Ian: The effects of dietary carbohydrate on high density lipoprotein levels in serum: Nutrition Reports Intl. Vol. 17. No. 6; 1978; pp663–68.
72. Howell, Edward: Enzyme Nutrition. Avery Pubshg: Njer 1985.
73. Taylor, Renee: Hunza Health Secrets. Keats Publishing. Conn. U.S.A. 1964.
74. Howell, Edward: Enzyme Nutrition. Avery. NJ. USA. 1985.
75. Ross, Harvey, M.: Fighting Depression: Larchmont Books, New York. 1975.
76. Turner, Roger Newman: Naturopathic Medicine: Thorsons 1990.
77. Int. J. Brit. Nutr. Res. 51, 232–238; 1981.
78. Coates, Dr. Nadyan, Jollyman, Norman: A Matter of Life; MacDonald & Co. 1990.
79. Adams, Ruth and Murray, Frank: Megavitamin Therapy; Lorchmont Book, New York. 1973.